Why Not Me?

Why Not Me?

The Power of Perspective

Lindsay Ireland

E. L. Marker
Salt Lake City

Published by E. L. Marker, an imprint of WiDo Publishing
Salt Lake City, Utah
widopublishing.com

This is a work of creative nonfiction. The events herein are portrayed to the best of the author's memory. While all the stories in this narrative are true, some names and identifying details may have been changed to protect the privacy of the people involved.

Cover design by Steven Novak
Book design by Marny K. Parkin

ISBN 978-1-947966-60-4

To my family

The idea behind a kaleidoscope is that it's a structure that's filled with broken bits and pieces, and somehow if you can look through them, you still see something beautiful. And I feel like we are all that way a little bit.

—Sara Bareilles

Author's note

Several names in this memoir have been changed to protect the privacy of certain individuals.

Contents

—ᴡᴡ—

Introduction

"Images of War"

—⟋⟍—

Sometimes I feel as if my body is a battlefield. That there have been wars fought on my belly, my ovaries and my brain. Over forty years have passed since I was admitted to The Hospital for Sick Children and, after much agony and confusion, was diagnosed with my first autoimmune disease.

The war images first started when I was at home recovering after my second surgery, when I caught a glimpse of myself in the mirror: at eleven years old I was sixty-five pounds with thinning hair and dark circles under my eyes. I immediately connected my reflection with the images I had seen of concentration camp victims. Death hadn't occurred to me consciously until that moment with the mirror.

I have come to terms with the external battle scars. I actually appreciate the outlook on life they have afforded me. The internal damage has been difficult to assess. Peace has been hard won by sifting through the rubble in my mind and evaluating the struggle with open eyes.

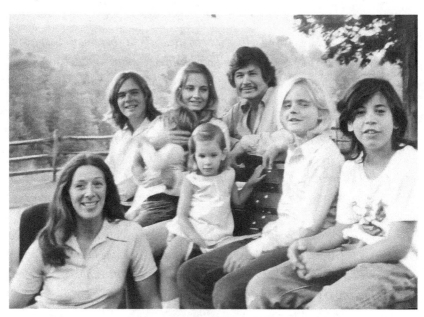

One of my first visits to Vermont. *From left:* Mum, Paul, Aunt Jill (Su on lap), Uncle Charlie, me, Val, and Jason. Summer, 1973.

Chapter 1

I like lemonade

—᠆᠆

"When they remain silent, they cry out."   —Marcus Tullius Cicero

To this day, I still feel like I am going home when I make the trip to Vermont. While many of my friends were attending summer camp, every August since I turned six my "campground" was at my Aunt Jill and Uncle Charlie's nineteenth-century horse farm called Sulika Farm in Vermont. This paradise consisted of 700 acres of wooded trails, two swimming ponds, and spacious rolling green horse paddocks surrounding their large, colonial style house. In the evening, when the horses were feeling frisky, my younger cousin and I were convinced that we could hear them calling us from our bedroom window.

With me in Vermont were my cousins Paul, Val, Jason, Tony, Suzanne, and Sulika, Su for short. Paul, Val, and Jason were like the older brothers I never had and playfully tormented Su and me when they weren't riding their dirt bikes. Tony and Suzanne were older, too, and were often with their mother for half the summer, so my time in Vermont didn't always overlap with theirs. My cousin Sulika and I were joined at the hip—I was two years her senior, but she was born August 4 and I was born August 8, so we spent our entire birth month together in Vermont. My sister, Courtenay, was still in diapers when I started making the trip to Vermont. She, Mum, and Dad stayed home while Dad grew his business and I got this special time with our relatives. This tradition continued until my teens.

My aunt and uncle were successful actors, but they didn't take any jobs during the summer months. They were able to spend their time freely and would be present around the farm each day. As kids, except for our daily riding lesson, Su and I occupied our time with various imaginative pursuits. Pretending that we were Nancy Drew and her sidekick George was our favourite activity. We spent hours building secret hideouts in the hayloft, or heroically searching for villains in the wooded trails accompanied by our trusty "guard dogs" Lucky Puppy and Fat Friday. With the dogs covered in mud and burrs, our matted hair and tanned, hay-scratched arms and legs, we made a motley foursome as we combed the property looking for clues to solve the mystery of the day.

On the days that we hung up our detective caps we fancied ourselves as adventurous explorers and, with Uncle Charlie's help, we would canoe the pond in search of rare wildlife. A successful hunt would yield a turtle-spotting, or the capture of a frog or toad. Heady stuff when you're a prepubescent adventurer-in-training. When we had found what we were looking for, we would take the long way home, with Uncle Charlie leading the way, picking the best route to cross streams and pick ripe blackberries.

Uncle Charlie was a famous actor, but to me, he was a man who enjoyed a good joke and saw the humour in life. Once, when Su and I were in our tween years, Uncle Charlie hid in the trees, by the back of the pond, making bear noises while Su and I were floating around on our inflatable loungers. We thought we were hearing things at first and went to sun ourselves on the dock. The "bear" was patient and made his noises sporadically. After about 30 minutes, our unease grew and we climbed into the nearby canoe to investigate.

While out paddling, we ventured close to the shore of the island and the growls grew increasingly louder; the incessant chirp of the crickets seemed to fade. The pond was always home to a symphony of sounds, but what usually felt like a familiar summer soundtrack of humming dragonflies, chirping crickets, jumping fish and croaking toads now felt ominous. Instead of a hot summer buzz, the air felt electric, full of tension. Our ears were focused on the noise of the bear. Was that him rustling. . . or was it the thrushes in the warm breeze?

Su and I were spooked and didn't want to walk back to the house. Just as we began assessing our escape options, Uncle Charlie leapt from behind a tree with a ferocious growl. He was grinning from ear to ear as our high-pitched shrieks pierced the air—I had to quickly rescue my paddle after I dropped it in fright. After taking a moment to calm our anxiety, and mildly chide him for scaring us, we laughingly relived his performance, and claimed we knew it was him all along. With our pride intact, and Uncle Charlie grinning like a Cheshire cat, we abandoned the canoe on the shore, and the three of us took the long way back to the house for lunch.

My uncle took immense pleasure out of day-to-day things, such as his walks in the woods and time with family. He was a man who didn't waste words. This might have made him seem aloof. I think he just didn't feel the need to fill dead air space, or to hear the sound of his own voice; he didn't enjoy engaging in small talk. He spoke up when it mattered and spent time with people he trusted. It took me a little while to figure that out and not be nervous around my uncle. Once I understood that aspect of his nature, I relaxed and respected his ways.

Aunt Jill spent a lot of time horseback riding, hanging out at the barn, or, when she was at the house, chatting on the phone and keeping up with correspondence. Some days she had a riding lesson with an older, Dutch, former Olympian named Dr. van Schaik. His manner and teaching style were very disciplined, and he was sought after for his effective instruction. Although his barn was a 40-minute drive, Aunt Jill didn't mind and would often bring us along for the trip. We would scramble into the passenger side of her two-seater, baby blue, 1965 Corvette convertible, singing songs with the warm air whooshing through our hair. I particularly liked when we sang a song that she had recorded for a movie that she and Uncle Charlie had filmed, *From Noon till Three.* The three of us knew all the words to "Hello and Goodbye" and would sing it loudly as we navigated the dirt roads in the summer heat. I felt carefree. Su and I would criss-cross our feet over each other's on the dash, covering the No Smoking sticker, while we linked arms. We shared the one seat belt; this was long before anyone cared much about car safety.

If we wanted to run the risk of getting lost, Aunt Jill would take us to a general store to buy a treat. Su always picked ice cream, and I would get lemonade. They both found my pick curious; to them, chocolate and ice cream were the obvious choices. It wasn't a mystery to me, I loved chocolate, but I was thirsty and wanted a sweet drink.

On many occasions, after driving away from the store, we'd return 10 minutes later and ask to use the phone. Aunt Jill needed Uncle Charlie to direct us home. Years later, I realized that, like me, my aunt had no internal GPS. Going places with her could often become an unintentional adventure.

Once in a while, Aunt Jill would take us for excursions to West Lebanon, a town about 30 minutes from the farm. We'd sometimes get our photo taken at JC Penney's, or she'd buy us matching t-shirts at Kmart. If Su and I had some of our own money, she'd drive us to the discount store, Rich's, to peruse the Barbie section. On rainy days, she and Uncle Charlie would take us to the movies. The boys were teenagers and usually did their own thing, but sometimes during the day, they joined us on the trampoline. On most days we'd see them zooming by, usually

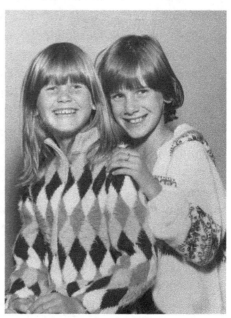

JC Penney portrait of Su and me. August, 1980.

with Uncle Charlie, disappearing into the woods on their dirt bikes, or they'd vanish to a friend's house to work on their music.

By 1980, I had been spending August in Vermont with Aunt Jill, Uncle Charlie, and my cousins for five years. My birthdays had developed into particularly momentous occasions because Sulika and I were born two years and four days apart. Aunt Jill and Uncle Charlie enjoyed sleeping in and luxuriating in their bed each day, and that

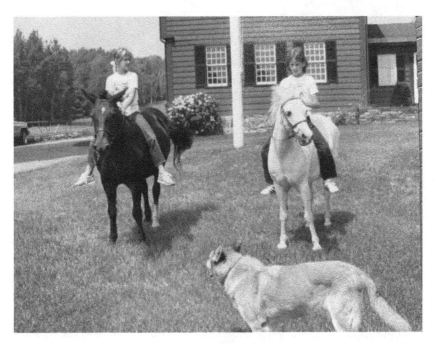

Su and me on ponies in Vermont. Summer, 1980.

included our birthdays, so we'd wait patiently before they'd appear to open our gifts.

On my 11th birthday, Su and I crept down to the living room on tippy toes, maneuvering the carpeted yet still creaky stairs carefully, to find two large (adult size!) suitcases covered in stickers and ribbon—there were red lips, gold hearts, bright rainbows and small gold stars plastered in an artistic pattern over the leather handle and blue canvas body of the luggage. Su's birthday was four days prior and she had awoken to the same scene, so I knew that these were not empty cases! They were jam-packed with gifts: crafts, clothes, games, Barbie doll items and hopefully a sweatshirt with my name on it, the only thing I had specifically requested. That year, I was very impressed by items that announced to the world who I was: LINDSAY. My last name was not important at the time, just LINDSAY. Aunt Jill didn't disappoint; I got my wish.

—⟋⟍—

It was that summer of 1980 when I first started having regular bouts of bloody diarrhea. The only clear memory I have of the blood is when Su and I interrupted an engrossing game of Nancy Drew we were playing at the Woodstock Inn—Aunt Jill and Uncle Charlie took us there for dinner—to take a bathroom break. We were wearing our matching smocked dresses and white leather sandals, and had been sleuthing around the hotel spying on the unsuspecting guests at the posh, New England establishment.

We chose to relieve ourselves in the hotel lobby ladies' room after taking a thorough snoop around the gift shop for potential thieves. I don't remember stomach pain or cramps but when I went to flush, I recall announcing "Nancy, there's blood in my poo."

Without missing a beat, Su replied "George, don't tell my mom or she'll make you go to the doctor."

I definitely did not want to be taken to the doctor, so I didn't mention the red streaks to anyone else. I spoke to my mum and dad each night on the telephone but didn't rate the news of my mysteriously streaked stool as worth mentioning. Maybe I didn't want my summer to end abruptly. It's more likely that I was ignorant about the serious causes of bloody stool, so was genuinely unconcerned. I wasn't slowing down, and Nancy and I had many more amusing capers to investigate. In retrospect, I think I was afraid of what might happen and that I would somehow be blamed.

I often worried about being blamed for things in Vermont. Aunt Jill and Uncle Charlie thought Su could do no wrong, and I would sometimes be held responsible for things we did together. Not big things, but, for example when we were both given Barbies, their coordinating outfits, and the Barbie Beauty Salon, Aunt Jill forbade us from opening our boxes before I went back to Toronto, less we mix up or lose the miniature shoes, combs, belts etc. . . Talk about dangling a carrot—the Barbie Carrot was more than the two of us could resist. I wasn't going home for over two weeks and we were itching to play with our new goods.

Su assured me that her mom wouldn't really mind—"She's try-ing to be tough," Su said. I wasn't so sure. Aunt Jill had looked very serious when she told us, but we went ahead with the plan to set up our salons and dress up our new dolls. We tore into those boxes with gusto. Just as we were making sure we didn't inadvertently toss any of Barbie's accessories into the trash, we looked up to see Aunt Jill, in her pale blue Reebok track suit, looming in the doorway. Her face was stern; she didn't like a mess and was obviously displeased. Su and I, knee-deep in Barbie boxes, sheepishly apologized.

Later in the day, while I was in Su's bedroom, which we shared, I heard Su and Aunt Jill whispering in the hall. Su was explaining that I had suggested we open all the toys so we could establish that there were no missing pieces. I wasn't surprised by this betrayal, but I sud-denly felt incredibly homesick and was desperate to talk to my mum. I needed to hear her voice.

That night in bed, when everyone should have been asleep, Aunt Jill snuck into our room and climbed into Su's four-poster bed for a cuddle beneath the sheets. Again, there was whispering—the mother-daughter snuggle was a nightly occurrence, but that night it made me feel more isolated than usual and I cried silently on my mattress on the floor.

Stifling distress was a habit I developed early in life. I was a kind, obedient child, and was insecure of my status as Su's play partner. I was nervous that my role might be revoked, and I'd be substituted by someone else. It was not until years later that I fully trusted that I was not a commodity to amuse Su, but family true and true.

A couple of weeks after my first abnormal bowel movement, I flew home to Toronto. I cried when I left Vermont, as I had when I left home to go to Vermont. Aunt Jill and Su drove me to Boston where we stopped to get my first manicure before they took me to the air-port. People used to get dressed up when they traveled and Aunt Jill made sure I was immaculately groomed for my flight. Aunt Jill had bought me a proper traveling outfit. I wore a forest green tunic, a white round-collared blouse and a Madeline-style felt hat. My spanking new black patent leather shoes made a distinct clicking sound as I approached the paunchy customs officer.

"Anything to declare?" he growled down his nose.

"Yes—I have a list my aunt wrote for you—she gave me presents and wrote them all down." I must have looked like a brat in my prissy getup but my hand was shaking as I produced my page of toys to declare.

His face softened and he stifled a chuckle while reviewing my impressive list of goodies. I guess the Barbie Beauty Parlour didn't warrant searching an 11-year-old. He told the stewardess accompanying me to make sure I found my parents safely. Maybe Aunt Jill had included an autographed photo of Uncle Charlie with the list? Maybe he could tell I wasn't the prig that my outfit suggested? Or possibly he wasn't accustomed to the honesty of Aunt Jill's list. It might just have been a bit of fun in his usually monotonous officious role. As for me, suffice to say, that is the one and only list I have ever handed over to a customs officer.

My mum and dad almost didn't recognize me when they collected me at the Toronto airport. I looked like a little lady instead of the farm ragamuffin I had been for the last month. It felt so good to see them again after a month apart. I'd missed them and was happy to be home. Su has been like a sister for the past month, but I couldn't wait to see Courtenay.

A few days before I was supposed to begin Grade 6, I was having cramps with my diarrhea and I showed my mum and dad the blood that I was passing. My dad raged on the phone to Aunt Jill to see what the hell I had been up to in Vermont. His temple was pulsing; I imagined his ears would start emitting smoke. My mum, seemingly calmer, took me to see our family doctor who promptly sent me to a pediatrician across the hall, who sent me to The Hospital for Sick Children (corporately branded as SickKids) for some tests.

It all happened so quickly. I was admitted to the isolation ward, which meant that anything I brought in, including books, stuffed animals, toys and clothes would not be able to leave when I did. I left my new LINDSAY sweatshirt at home, although, in hindsight, it would have been an appropriate time to keep my identity in full view. Only my parents, nurses and doctors were allowed in my room, and they all wore scrubs, gloves and covers on their shoes. This garb was to protect them from me. Was I poison?

The door to my room remained closed at all times and I had to press a button to summon a nurse, the warden of this prison. Pressing the button would activate a red light in the hallway over the door to the antiseptic cell. It was all so quiet, like the calm before the storm. Like in the movies when your heart starts quickening because you know something is going to make you jump, so you hold your breath in anticipation. It's a wonder my lungs didn't burst.

Chapter 2

Bedside stories

—ᕽᕽᕽ—

"We're all a little fragile."   —Kiran Shaiki

During my time in isolation, the cramps in my abdomen drastically increased, and so did the blood that I was passing with my stool. My health continued to deteriorate, but seemingly, I wasn't contagious. Five days after being admitted, I was released from the infectious disease ward and placed in a normal hospital room. One of my roommates had asthma, the other, cancer.

I didn't know what I had, but I don't recollect being particularly curious as to what was ailing me. Maybe I wasn't a kid who asked "why" all the time, or maybe the prospective answer terrified me. My theory is that I was too tired and weak to care. I was shell-shocked from the pain and drugs and didn't think much of anything. Usually a voracious reader, I lacked the energy for books and fell in and out of sleep watching TV. The hospital machines and hallways could be noisy, so I enjoyed the quiet when it came.

After almost three weeks of being bedridden, the doctors thought I should try and get out of bed to take a short walk. Even if it was just down the hospital corridor, it sounded like a good idea to me. Maybe I was progressing? I liked the idea of getting out of bed and onto my feet again. Maybe I could use a toilet instead of the cold metal bedpan? Mum and Dad kept assuring me that I would get better and go home. Maybe this would literally be a step in that direction.

The nurse found a wheelchair, I was lifted into it, and all my IV bags were put onto one pole. Mum pushed me into the hallway. It was longer and narrower than I had envisioned with a big window at the end. My goal was to go have a look out the window. Seeing the outside world again was enormously appealing. The world of my hospital room was small, and my bed even more confining.

They locked the chair wheels, and Mum and the nurse helped lift me to a standing position. I leaned into them as I attempted to steady myself to take my first steps. My legs buckled. Without their assistance I would have crashed to the floor. There was no hope that I was walking that morning, I couldn't even stand up. I had not been expecting that defeat. I knew I was sick, but I assumed I could still walk. The entire exercise of getting out of bed, into the chair, standing up and collapsing had exhausted me. I was taken back to bed, the bedside rails raised and I asked for my next painkiller. I cried as I waited for the injection of Demerol.

—⚉—

The days all blended into one another and I had no reason or enough energy to be concerned about time. A central line had been surgically implanted in my neck to feed me. I was really skinny, but hadn't seen myself since I left home, so I didn't know how skeletal I was. I was a thin girl to start with and I didn't have any extra fat to lose.

It quickly became apparent that I was now too sick to be in a semi-private room. My vital stats were being taken every 20 minutes, which wasn't conducive for good sleeping, but I'd been told it was necessary due to my depleted body weight, blood loss and the high doses of prednisone that were being used to treat me. I hadn't been out of bed again for about two weeks when I was wheeled down the hall to a private room with a private nurse, Cindy. It was like being in an intensive care unit (ICU), but on a regular ward.

Cindy was new to nursing and I was her first patient, so we had something in common—we were both new to our roles. She was young, tall, and pretty, with short blonde hair. She had a soothing voice and didn't rush around like some of the other nurses. Cindy wasn't slow, but she did things like they mattered. I felt like I mattered. I have met and been cared for by many, many, good nurses in hospital, but hers is the only name I remember.

Cindy spoiled me. She was not only kind and caring; she gave me little gifts. I'm not sure why they stuck her with such a sickie on her first week but I knew I had won the Nurse Lottery. My parents loved her because she was so good to me. On my second day with Cindy she gave me a hand-knit grey mouse in a red gingham dress to tie to the end of my steel bed rails. Mousie watched over me on days when Cindy was off; she felt like my guardian angel with her serene stitched look.

—ᴍ—

My mum and dad took turns staying with me and slept in a big blue leather La-Z-Boy chair in my room. My sister didn't see much of our parents during this time. Mum arranged a favourite family babysitter for Courtenay, or for her to go to various friend's houses after school, until she could be picked up by Mum or Dad. Court remembers liking going to some houses more than others, and feeling relieved when she could stay home with the babysitter.

Whenever I woke up, I would see either Mum or Dad in that chair, on guard for me. I don't remember what Mum and I talked about all those days that she sat there beside me. I do remember that she had a very distinct pattern to her walk, and I always knew when it was her coming down the hall in the morning. I was enormously comforted by her clicking sound. It was only about a two-hour gap from when Dad left in the very early morning until when Mum arrived, but my ear was attuned for her appearance. Mum usually did the day shift and made sure that I always had a clean hospital gown or nightie. She once bought me a pink one, patterned with colourful hearts, that tied at the shoulders to make it easier to get on and off over my IV's.

Every day, after my bed bath, which resulted in soggy sheets, Mum or Dad and the nurse made up my bed with me in it. If you haven't experienced this, it's quite a feat. To change the bedding, I was gingerly rolled from side to side while the bedding was stripped. At this point, if I had been a package I would have been marked "FRAGILE— Handle with Care." My body was all bone. Had I been able to stand up and hug someone, my ribs would have punctured them. When my old sheets were removed, clean ones were laid out with the same method of them rolling me from side to side until the bed was made. They always found whatever flannel sheets were stashed in the ward's linen cupboard to keep me warm.

Dad would stay overnight so that he could continue to manage the printing company that he owned. He was usually very occupied with his business, while Mum got me and my sister ready for the day, volunteered at our school and read to us at night. I remember many late-night chats with my father during this period. It was the first time in my life that I had spent big chunks of time talking alone with him.

Without work to distract him, he told me about how he learned to swim (his dad threw him in the freezing English sea), what he and his "mates" got up to (no good) and the first time he ever tasted Coca Cola—Dad was 14, and had just played a game of football (English soccer) when someone presented him with a glass bottle of Coke. He said he had never tasted anything so divine, that it was a sweet nectar coating his throat. During my first time in hospital, I learned more about my family by the light of my Total Parenteral Nutrition (TPN) IV drip than ever before.

My dad, John Ireland, was born in Hounslow, England in 1939 to Jack and Dorothy Ireland, and was two and a half years younger than his sister Jill. Both children were good-looking, outgoing, lively and animated. Jill was blonde with blue eyes, and loved to dance. Dad had brown eyes, dark hair, an elfin grin, and was constantly on the move. Grandpa managed a grocery store, and the family was lower middle class. Things were tight financially, but there was always enough to get by. They lived with the post-war mentality that nothing was wasted. Dad recalls using congealed bacon fat as butter on his toast. None of them ever thought to complain about any shortages; everyone they knew was in the same boat.

At a young age, Aunt Jill and Dad were both involved in the performing arts. Grandma was a stage mother long before Kris (Kardashian) Jenner took the term to another level. Dad was a child actor with a troupe who travelled Europe staging Shakespearean plays. He also won small parts in movies. His sister was primarily a dancer who got bit-acting parts on the stage. Years later, she told me that when she watched her brother on stage, she was intensely jealous of his natural acting ability. He was good. He received excellent reviews for his work in the local papers.

Acting was a terrific outlet for his natural desire for the limelight. Dad's ability to command attention in a crowd is something that I admire. Even before I got sick, I was exceptionally shy as a child and my fear of public speaking never got easier for me. Dad comes by it naturally. In later life, Dad's nickname at his golf club was Hollywood John. He was frequently asked to emcee events and address the crowd at tournaments. Growing up, Dad thrived in social situations, but his mischievous nature got him into trouble more and more. Jill got most of the positive attention at home.

As a teenager, Dad's mother enrolled him in acting school where he did well. This was interrupted when he was seventeen and called up for an army physical. He missed an important audition for *Hamlet* that day, but luckily, he missed more than that. The physical revealed a large mastoid in his left ear, and he was exempted from the Armed Forces.

The competition for acting parts was becoming fierce, and traveling with an all-male cast was proving to be lonely, so he put aside his love of acting, and got a job at a local news outlet as a cub reporter, collecting news clips at the London airport. The job paid very little, so he quickly moved up to an office role as a typographer. He spent the next six years at this job and going out socializing with his friends in the evening. He was popular and had a broad circle of chums, but was also prone to getting into scraps at bars. He and Aunt Jill shared some friends, although she shied away from the ruffian types, as she was trying to make her mark as a serious performer. By age sixteen, she had earned spots in several successful chorus lines and was performing at the Hippodrome and Palladium in London.

In 1957, Aunt Jill married a fellow actor, David McCallum. They were forging successful career paths in England and, watching their careers take off, my grandma began to worry that Dad's antics with his buddies might soil my aunt's reputation. As Aunt Jill and David became more visible publicly, the family wanted Dad to become less so. In the spring of 1962, Grandma, Grandpa and Aunt Jill asked Dad to move to Canada to create some distance from Jill's increasingly high-profile London life. Canada was seen as the land of opportunity, so with $50 in his pocket, Dad did as he was asked and booked a ticket on the *Empress of England* and set sail for the next chapter of his life.

When I learned why Dad came to Canada, feelings I had from my childhood came into focus. I had sensed that my dad's mum valued Aunt Jill's side of the family more than ours. Grandma and Grandpa had been in Vermont during my first summer visit there. I became aware that Grandma had sent Su special gifts. Su had innocently showed Grandma where she kept her presents in front of me. They were things to make a young girl feel special; I remember a shiny silver beaded purse and a china cat figurine. I had never received such treasures from England. Courtenay was just a baby at this point, but nothing extraordinary had ever arrived for her either. I felt hurt and confused, but didn't dwell on it. I needed my grandparents on that trip.

I think that first summer in Vermont was a test run to measure my compatibility for Su. I slept in a guest room with Grandma and Grandpa, on a cot between their single beds. Grandma had equipped me with a long, empty, cardboard wrapping paper roll, and given me the important job of whacking Grandpa on the head whenever he snored in the night. Luckily for Grandpa, I didn't have any violent tendencies, and he was very good-natured about the mild abuse. I have a feeling Grandma would have liked me to hit him harder, but she always playfully smiled as she praised me for doing an excellent job. I was enveloped in my grandparents' presence, and our little blue and white room felt cozy and filled with good humour. If we were having a lazy morning and moving slowly, Su would come to our room to make sure we joined her for breakfast. The four of us would end up chatting while we lolled around on the little beds. I enjoyed those times. Near the end of my stay that summer, I had a sleepover in my younger cousin's room and that did it—I moved my things to her closet the next day and our summer visits properly began.

Much later in my life, I felt very grateful for the fact that Su had been born two years after me, and that we shared the same birth month. I realized that she and I became the main reason for Dad and Aunt Jill to reconnect as siblings. I recently found a letter that Aunt Jill had written to Grandma, Grandpa and my parents after she had come to England with two-year-old Su to visit us while we were there on vacation. She hadn't seen my dad, her brother, since he had left for Canada almost seven years earlier. She enjoyed seeing Dad, meeting Mum, and thought that I was a good influence on Su. Also, she wrote that her daughter was clearly taken with me. That was the start of what became a very important family connection. At first, it was just me going to Vermont in the summers, but later we started having family Christmases there too.

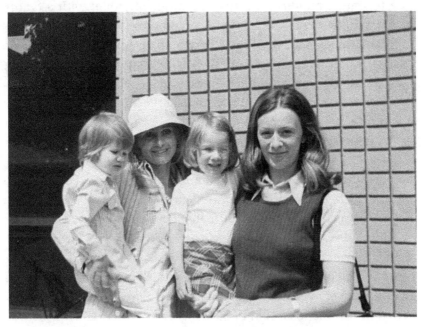

Su, Aunt Jill, me, and Mum meeting for the first time at Heathrow airport. 1973.

My mother, Sandra Hawthorne, had taken the train from her hometown of Paisley, near Glasgow, Scotland, and boarded the same ship the very day my dad embarked. She thought she would visit Canada for a while to get some distance from her overbearing mother, while having a bit of an adventure. She didn't plan on making Canada home.

Like me, Mum was the eldest of two children. She was born in November 1940, sixteen months before her brother Gordon. Gordon had been a twin and his sister had died shortly after birth. Unfortunately, Grandma would bring this up repeatedly over the years, suggesting to Mum, "If Catherine had lived, she would be here to help me." This was just one line in her arsenal of unkind guilt trips.

Uncle Gordon was a spirited little boy who had no interest in rules. Mum was the opposite. She was an anxious child who towed the line. I could relate to that. When she was young, her family lived in a tenement building and shared an outside toilet with a family of five adults. Mum was terrified of going to the toilet at night in the dark. When she was done, she would remain in the blackness, perched on the seat, peering out the keyhole, frozen in fright, waiting for her dad to come and walk her back to their flat.

From five years old, Mum was an avid reader and therefore, very aware of the resources that her family lacked. She lost herself in books about affluent girls in boarding schools, who had their own horses. The smell of leather saddles, boots and barns practically floated off the pages and she would become spellbound by that fantasy world. My summers in Vermont must have seemed idyllic to her. It was an opportunity she only dreamed of as a child.

Mum's dad, Bill Hawthorne, was the more loving, gentle parent than Mum's mum. He made Mum feel treasured. Papa was an engine fitter and money was tight. Grandma worked at menial jobs during the first 20 years of their marriage to augment the family finances. When Mum was fourteen, Papa contracted tuberculosis and was hospitalized for eighteen months and Grandma's income became their sole means of support. Mum did her part to help out by leaving school at fifteen and secured a clerking job in a Glasgow office. Mum loved school and would have preferred to continue her education but felt obliged to get a job as Gordon was attending high school and manfully doing an early morning milk delivery before school as well as a paper route after school.

Even now, I think Mum still feels, and laments, the sting of her poor childhood. Having less than most of her grammar school classmates has left faded, but still present, scar tissue. I think the shame and fear that she experienced regarding her family financial situation may be similar to the post-traumatic shock emotions I felt regarding my ill health. They can leave nasty imprints on your psyche. Later in life, I successfully dulled those through therapy. Instead of just feeling lucky to have a financial cushion, I also feel grateful to be alive.

When Mum's mum was six years old, her mother died of pneumonia and she was cared for by her paternal grandmother. This much-loved grandmother died when Grandma was thirteen years old, and she was then cared for by her two aunts, Milly and Bessie, who she referred to as her sisters. My middle names Elizabeth and Amelia are in honour of those women who played a large role in the lives of Mum and Grandma. The family dynamics left my grandma with feelings of inferiority and self-pity which she never overcame. This did not result in her being timid—quite the opposite—she was bossy and an attention hog. She was an intelligent, attractive blonde, had a good figure, and often flirted with men for attention.

Knowing what we know now, Grandma might have been bipolar. She could be fun, hilariously funny, and make you feel like the centre of the universe, and then, in the next breath be cuttingly distant and mean. She suffered a nervous breakdown when Mum was in her thirties and was hospitalized for months. This was long before talking about mental health was fashionable, or encouraged, so her time away was a bit of a mystery. Mum, Gordon and Papa felt the warm glow when Grandma shone her spotlight on them, but also put up with some crazy and cruel behaviours. Papa managed by keeping quiet and disappearing to the dog racetracks, Gordon ended up an alcoholic, and Mum escaped to Canada.

Mum and Dad met on the *Empress of England*. The ship set sail from Liverpool on April 18, 1962 and was bound for Montreal. Mum was alluring with her bright blue eyes, long, thick, dark brown hair, pretty face and perfectly proportioned curves. She was a good girl who was quick to laugh and enjoyed a good time, and was attracted to Dad's sense of humour and amusing anecdotes. He was handsome, charming and entertaining.

When they arrived at the railway station in Toronto, Aunt Jill's friend from home, Jim Heather, met Dad. Looking dashing in his MG sports car, Jim arrived to whisk Dad off to the newly acquired apartment that he shared with his wife, Margaret. Dad gave Jim's phone number to Mum so they could stay connected. Mum found accommodations with two other women from the ship. Mum and Dad kept in touch, and soon began dating. They spent a lot of time with Jim and Margaret as well as one of Mum's roommates, Joan. Without any other family or friends in Canada, they all became each other's family, and later, mine too. Dad was not in a rush to be married, but Mum wanted to make things official, so she convinced him that settling down was a good idea. Just less than two years after landing in Canada, they planned a small wedding, with only their new friends in attendance.

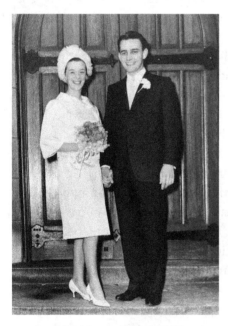

Mum and Dad on their wedding day. February 2, 1964.

Years later, when I was in hospital, "Uncle Jim" visited me almost every day after work. The nurses sometimes mistook him for my dad. They had the same English accent, sense of humour, and looked very similar. Connecting Dad with Jim may have been Aunt Jill's biggest gift to her brother; they became the best of friends. It's been years since Uncle Jim died, but Aunt Margaret is still an important part of our family.

When Mum and Dad were first married, they bought a house on a farm outside of Toronto. In keeping with their modest means, it was a fixer-upper of a house and barn, and although they didn't have two nickels to rub together, they owned two horses. Mum was mucking her own stalls, but she achieved her dream for a while, and loved it. I was born while they lived on the farm and Mum would take me in my bassinet to sleep on the hay bales while she cleaned up after the horses. Maybe those early smells account for my love of horses to this day.

Mum came to Canada knowing she had a job secured as a secretary, and Dad quickly found work selling printing equipment. Mum missed the relative glamour of her secretarial job at Scottish Television, and had no career aspirations. She worked to pay the bills. If she didn't feel like going in to work, she would call in sick and spend the day in bed reading. She was mostly a good employee though; her fingers flew over the typewriter; she was very literate and quick with numbers. Her boss wasn't shy in hitting on her, which at the time wasn't a big deal, many men didn't seem to know any better.

Dad quickly became one of the printing company's top salesmen. I have a feeling that with his charisma, humour and looks, Dad could have sold ice to polar bears, and with his employment background, energy, and solid work ethic, he was the real deal. He was the Energizer Bunny, always planning ahead and ambitious. He was like that my whole life.

When I was two, my parents sold the farm and moved to the city. After making a good living selling printing presses, Dad started his own printing company. He ended up with printing contracts for the flyers, catalogues and newspaper inserts for the big-name Canadian department stores. As Dad's business grew my parents upgraded their houses.

Chapter 3

I'm getting a rosebud?

—ɯɯ—

"What we have in common with the rosebud, which trembles because a drop of dew is lying upon it?" —Friedrich Nietzsche

I have some vivid memories from hospital and then there are entire episodes where I must have changed the channel, because I haven't the vaguest notion of how the story goes. During my time on prednisone, my health continued to rapidly deteriorate. My aunt Jill and Su came to stay with my mum, dad and Courtenay. I remember when Aunt Jill arrived at the hospital. She glowed, wearing a red parachute jumpsuit, silver padded vest, silver sneakers and a diamond brooch on the neck of her jumpsuit that spelled LOVE. She sailed into my room—it was as if someone turned a light on. Su was right behind her; she looked the same as when I had left her a month earlier, tanned and healthy. I don't remember them kissing me hello, but they likely did. They stood beside my bed, animatedly talking while they clasped my bed rails.

Aunt Jill prattled on, "The boys, Suzanne and Uncle Charlie say hi and are worried about you. They send their love. The horses and dogs miss you too. I think Fat Friday is looking for you. Su and Champ did well in a horse show last week. It wasn't as fun for me without you there as my show buddy . . ."

Su interrupted "Yeah, Mom missed you for sure. Champ was amazing and we aced the cross country. We have another show next week. I don't collect the empty bottles without you, so haven't been making any money for going to Rich's."

I smiled. Between Su's horse show events, she and I would scour the area near the food stands for empty pop cans and return them for cash. Sometimes we'd find the odd beer bottle too. It was a great way to fill dead time and make some money for Barbie clothes. We were still sleuthing, just with some financial purpose.

During their visit, I saw how my cousin and aunt were so full of life. Mum had lost 15 pounds, and she and Dad had dark circles etched under their eyes. It looked like my deterioration was killing them too, although they always managed to be strong, immensely caring and positive for me. Aunt Jill was a breath of fresh air, in sharp contrast to my parents.

With my mum in tow, Aunt Jill and Su disappeared from my hospital room to the Eaton Centre on the afternoon of their arrival. They weren't gone for long and reappeared with the newly released Barbie dog, a tape cassette of the movie soundtrack to *Grease,* and a portable tape deck. Su and I had been singing *Grease* songs all summer and we fancied ourselves as the Sandy character. Olivia Newton-John was our idol. And John Travolta was the coolest of the cool. That man was my heartthrob. When I see him on the screen now, I wonder where did his wiry body and slinky hips disappear to?

Seeing Aunt Jill and Su at the hospital was a great distraction and reminded me of all our adventures in Vermont. Nancy Drew wasn't going to solve my medical mystery, but Su's active imagination and upbeat prattle kept me thinking about the fun times in Vermont, how much I loved my time there, and when I'd get to go back.

Aunt Jill and Uncle Charlie were happiest in Vermont, away from the superficial and materialistic lifestyle they were surrounded by in Los Angeles. In Windsor, Vermont, they were Jill and Charlie, but in Bel Air, Los Angeles, they were Jill Ireland and Charles Bronson, the movie stars. Fame followed them everywhere, but their life was more centered on the family, farm and outdoors when they were in Vermont. There were no gala dinners to attend, no Neiman Marcus (or Needless Markup, as Aunt Jill fondly referred to it), and few autograph-seeking tourists. For my Uncle Charlie, the more reclusive of the two, Vermont was his haven. As a member of the family, I was fortunate to enjoy this retreat.

I didn't really grasp how famous Uncle Charlie was until I was in my teens. People born after 1980 will likely have to google Charles Bronson, but he was a big deal in his day. When we were in town, people sometimes stared and whispered his name, or asked him for his autograph, but usually, in Vermont, people weren't too intrusive. The locals were used to his presence. We would drive to town in a practical Ford Bronco SUV, and we blended in, as it was an unassuming vehicle favoured by many in the area.

In the early seventies, Uncle Charlie was a number one box office draw, commanding $1 million per film. This was more than most actors at that time. He was craggy-faced, rugged, and simmered with an underlying intensity on screen. He usually played tough guys and exuded strength on film, and in real life. Some people called him ugly, others good-looking. Nobody could say that his face didn't have tremendous character. To me, he was just Uncle Charlie and I loved it when he smiled and his eyes twinkled. There aren't many photos of him like this, but just because they weren't recorded on film doesn't mean it didn't happen often.

Uncle Charlie co-starred in Hollywood classics such as *The Magnificent Seven* (1960), *The Great Escape* (1963), and *The Dirty Dozen* (1967). His list of film credits is long, and he was a huge star in Europe and Asia, but it was not until 1974 when he starred in the vigilante film *Death Wish* that his status as a leading man in the US was solidified. That movie spawned four sequels during the seventies and eighties and secured him big pay checks going forward.

The Great Escape was the movie that changed his life in another lasting way. He met my aunt Jill. She was a beautiful, blonde, English actress fifteen years his junior. They were both married at the time, with kids. It started out as a friendship, but there was an intense attraction between them. A couple of years later, the magnetic pull was too strong to resist any longer. They both divorced their spouses, and in 1968 Aunt Jill and Uncle Charlie married and blended their families; my aunt had three young boys, Paul, Val and Jason, and my uncle had a son and a daughter, Tony and Suzanne. A few years later Sulika was born, their only biological child together.

—⟁—

While Aunt Jill was in town, after about two weeks in my private room, I learned that I had been diagnosed with ulcerative colitis (UC). I don't think anyone directly told me of this diagnosis, but I learned most things by listening to the doctors speak, amongst themselves, or to my parents. At age eleven, and in my depleted state, no one told me the ins and outs of UC or that it causes inflammation and ulcers in the colon and rectum.

I have since learned from my parents that a surgeon had visited me once when I was in the shared hospital room. His name was Dr. Filler and he was Chief of Surgery—he had reassured my parents, "I'm just checking on Lindsay, don't worry about my title." As I got sicker, Dr. Filler followed my case more closely with my gastroenterologist and eventually he had a meeting in a private room with my parents. At the time, I wasn't aware of the devasting dialogue that took place between them. When I asked, Mum shared it with me years later.

Dr. Filler ushered my parents to a small room down the hall from the nurse's station. He closed the door to give the three of them some privacy. There wasn't much need for opening chit chat, my parents knew they were there to talk about my situation. Dr. Filler explained, "Lindsay is losing blood faster than we can replace it."

I'd received a lot of blood transfusions during this time. It struck me as strange to have so many strangers' blood pulsing through my body, but because it was supposed to help me, it seemed sort of amazing, not gross. Mum asked, "What about the blood transfusions?" She had been hopeful that, with time, the extra blood would stabilize me.

Dr. Filler said, "We can't restore the ongoing depletion of vital minerals and electrolytes, including potassium. The risk is that very low levels of potassium can cause the heart to stop."

Mum and Dad were processing this when Dr. Filler mentioned the he was worried that my colon might also rupture. There was no good news, but neither of my parents wanted me cut open. Grasping at straws, my mum asked, "What about the steroid treatments?"

"It is very clear that the steroid treatments aren't working and the waiting period for an improvement is over" replied Dr. Filler. He could see my parents were devasted by the idea of me undergoing the knife. He pressed on, "Mr. and Mrs. Ireland, it is now a life-or-death situation. Without the intervention of ostomy surgery, I cannot be responsible for her life."

With that statement, my parents understood; deflated, they relented. There was no choice, they agreed to the surgery. At the time, I didn't know I was on death's door, but I'm sure it's why my aunt Jill showed up. She and Su also paid some much-needed attention to Courtenay during this dark time.

The day after my parents signed off on the surgery, an enterostoma nurse named Pat Fivey came to visit me to draw a circle about the size of a silver dollar on my stomach in red pen. I remember her voice, but not exactly what she said. She had short hair, was makeup-free, wore glasses, and had a calm voice and warm smile. Her nature didn't match her actions as she placed a cold metal 4 × 4 template by my belly button with several size circular cut-outs. Pat chose the 1½ inch circle and traced it on my body. Had my body become a canvas? It was already a pincushion for the nurses and a teaching instrument for the residents, but a drawing board for this lady named Pat? She didn't even look artistic! I didn't ask any questions as she drew and talked. I was dumbfounded by this mysterious artiste/nurse.

Later I learned this circle was where I was going to get a plastic bag on my stomach. My dad explained to me that I was going to be undergoing an operation to cut out my diseased colon (large intestine), and this would result in a bag on my stomach to collect my stool.

I remember I was confused about what the bag would be like, but I was too sick to ask questions or understand its significance. I was just getting through one hour to the next. I don't think my dad fully understood its significance either, even though his dad has had a colostomy. I do remember being advised by Pat, that where the circle was drawn was going to be the location of my stoma. A stoma? Never heard of it. She said the stoma would look like a red rosebud. A rose on my stomach? That was a bewildering prospect to say the least. The picture on my screen fades here, too much static. . . . I don't know what was going on in my doped-up brain.

The next morning the hospital Chaplin came by my room. We didn't request a visit, so when I saw the man with the white collar pop his head in, I remember thinking "this must be serious." It was just me and Mum in the room and neither of us were comforted by his presence. I was perplexed, but Mum seemed angered by this man of the cloth. He kindly asked if he could help in any way. Mum asked "Can you explain why God would allow this type of suffering for a child."

His reply was, "God only gives these challenges to those who can handle them."

I was thinking "Ah, come on, that can't be right" while Mum gave the slightest of eye rolls.

The Chaplin was there to provide comfort, but all he did was remind me of the last rites that I had seen on television. Even so, I didn't consciously worry about death. He didn't stay long, and again, I asked no questions. This wasn't because I was stupid, I was just a kid and my faith was in my parents to take care of me, not in a God I knew nothing about. When he left, I caught a few moments of sleep until my vitals were taken again.

A few hours later, a 16-year-old girl came to visit me to assure me that life would be dandy after I had a "bag." The ileostomy, more commonly referred to as a bag, would not mean that I couldn't wear swimsuit or tight clothes, and to demonstrate this point she had worn jeans that were painted on. She had just come back from Florida with some friends and had a fabulous week of sun'n'fun.

I was withering away in my hospital bed and had no idea what Miss Perky Pants was talking about. I thought, what is an ileostomy? Why am I supposed to care? I am going to have a garbage bag welded to my stomach, or so I thought. I was left feeling baffled, but I later learned that the slim, trim, healthy young visitor was successful in lifting Mum's spirits.

I didn't utter a single word during the visit—I hadn't a clue what to say.

—⚌—

When I look back on this time, it seems like I was set up to feel fear and shame about my ostomy. In 1980, there was no internet. My mum and dad were trying to collect information from the Encyclopedia. Why didn't the hospital staff just show me a bag? The visitor girl could of too. It would have demystified the situation and my imagination wouldn't have had as much space to roam. As an adult, if I've helped someone who is about to get an ostomy, I ask them if they would like to see mine. They always say "yes." It's a simple and a quick viewing. I pull down the waist band of my pants and underwear a few inches and they get the idea of what's ahead for them. This demonstrates my openness and instead of just seeing how easy it is to hide the bag in clothes they also see that I'm not ashamed of the bag; it's not some monstrosity to hide. It took me years to be comfortable to share my bag with others, even when I knew just seeing me clothed might be helpful. As a kid, I was once asked to be a "support visitor" and felt faint as I entered the hospital ward. I never tried again. I felt safer keeping my ostomy private, invisible. I did this for so long that I allowed my true self to be invisible too.

The Chaplin and teenager were the extent of the emotional preparations that my parents and I received pre surgery. The next morning, the clinical preparations continued—the nurse came to wash my belly with iodine, attach a new monitoring device, and insert another IV. Once the nurse's tasks were completed, she advised the waiting orderly that I was "ready to go."

Chapter 4

Smells like death

—ᴍ—

"Scars are simply modern battle wounds. Sometimes the enemy happens to be inside us." —Andrew Grey

I was wheeled down to surgery in my metal hospital bed with Mum, Dad and Aunt Jill following behind in a single file line. It was like a macabre game of Follow the Leader. We all squished in to the Patients Only elevator and were quiet as we made our way to the surgical floor. My family kept me company in the pre-surgical waiting area and stood around me chatting away the time. Their three voices felt like home to me, especially their English and Scottish accents. Home felt far away so it didn't really matter what they were saying, just that they were there. I did my best to listen and didn't say much.

No one was wearing bright colours that day, it was all neutrals. Mum and Aunt Jill hadn't bothered with lipstick; I guess bright and cheery hadn't been on their morning make-up menu. We were the only ones in the bland, badly lit room, and there was nothing interesting to look at except each other. The three of them held on to me through my bed railings as we waited for the nurse to come and roll me to the operating room. I don't think they wanted to let go for fear I would disappear. To keep the mood light, we chuckled about Aunt Jill's attempt to cook dinner the week before, resulting in green stew. After years of employing a cook at home, Aunt Jill didn't have a knack for meal preparations but she wanted to be helpful. Su had delighted in the meal because it reminded her of Dr. Seuss's story *Green Eggs and Ham*.

We were interrupted when the nurse came to wheel me away. I said goodbye to Mum, Dad and Aunt Jill. I didn't cry. I was taken down a long narrow corridor with several people passing by in doctor's scrubs of green pajama pants, coordinating short sleeve tops and patterned cotton caps. I was steered into a large bright room. It smelled of iodine, Lysol and antiseptic. I remember noticing that the operating room was silver and white, cold and quiet. The effect was eerie. I yearned in silence for my flannel PJ's, cozy bed and Siamese cat, Suki.

They slid me onto a narrow stainless-steel bed. It felt like I was being served up on a silver tray. I was a Thanksgiving turkey and the next step would be the carving. The light above me was huge and blinding. It took me a while to focus and register my surroundings. To the right side of my head, at eye level, was a small steel table on wheels with an array of scalpels and scissors. The tools were lying on what seemed to be a green dishcloth that matched the doctors' outfits in the hall. As soon as I registered the sight of the instruments, I turned my line of vision back to the enormous steel ceiling light. Better to be blinded than think too much about the role of the scalpel.

The room felt cold and even smelled cold. I imagined that this place was very similar to a morgue, with bodies being preserved in a cool climate. The nurse placed a warm blanket on me so I didn't shiver.

"How did you get the blanket so hot?" I wondered out loud.

"We put them in a dryer, sweetie."

She's either thoughtful or going to suffocate me with the warm cotton, I thought. I wasn't sure whom to trust in a room that easily fit my idea of a death chamber.

A clear plastic mask was placed over my mouth and I was told to breathe deeply because this would put me to sleep. I didn't question this instruction because in my heart I felt that sleep sounded like a very pleasant release from the terror that was setting in from my head to my toes. When I wake up will this bad, bad dream be over? I breathed in, smelled onions, tasted garlic and drifted away.

Hours later, when I grudgingly regained consciousness, my stomach felt heavy and sore; the pain sensation made me wonder if my belly was in a sort of vice grip and someone had placed a cement slab over the pinched flesh. I heard strangers talking but they sounded very far away. Was I in a tunnel? The voices came closer.

"Lindsay, open your eyes."

I blinked.

"Come on now, look at me, we have to roll you over, hon."

No way, José.

"Lindsay, we have nice heated blankets to put behind your back but we have to roll you over."

Heated blankets, well, ok . . . just get rid of your bullhorn and stop shouting at me. I squinted my eyes and it was like I was looking through warped binoculars. I saw that the recovery area was a long institutional-like room and beside me was a little boy crying in his cage of a bed. His sobs made me feel helpless and melancholy. In slow motion, my voice requested that the nurse try to help him stop crying; she thought the noise was bothering me.

I wasn't complaining, and so I painstakingly managed to make my fuzzy mouth form the words "I feel bad for him . . . so sad." I knew if I cried it would hurt, so I released myself back into the blackness of sleep.

Chapter 5

6C

—⟋⟍—

"It's not the bite of the snake that kills you, it's the poison left behind."
—Tom Callos

I woke up in my new room in Ward 6C and the first thing I registered was a life-size hot pink plastic hand on a spring waving back and forth in my face. What a trip! The hand was on a suction cup attached to my bed railing and there was a message inscribed on the palm. I couldn't focus to read it. I recognized my aunt's distinctive script, but couldn't make out the words.

Mum and Dad were there to see my eyes open and tell me that I was okay, and that the hand was a message from Aunt Jill, who had gone back to Vermont. She had written that she loved me, to get well soon and that she would send me some Calvin Klein jeans and Little Hero track suits. Next, I noticed three, 5-inch tall, clip-on, cartoon characters made of felt hugging my IV pole. Su had found them in the gift shop. Bugs Bunny, Sylvester the cat and Daffy Duck were now smiling down on me from below my bags of fluid and medications. I forced a smile and tried to talk, but couldn't seem to open my mouth to make the words come out. My body ached for another painkiller. My mind was working in slow motion, but my brain was alive enough to be silently pleading "Mum, Dad, help, it hurts. Please, please, please, help me. Ow." All I could muster was "It hurts."

I have no idea how many hours later I woke up again. My mum was sitting in the chair beside my bed and the moment she saw my eyes open, she came to attention and reached for my hand. After squeezing Mum's hand, I noticed a nurse standing over me with one of those kidney-shaped plastic hospital basins in her hand. I reckoned that it might make a nice hot tub for Barbie . . . I'll have to bring one home. Mid-Barbie thought, I expanded my sight line down to include my belly. The view was shocking. God help me! What is that squished, bloody, red hunk of flesh on my belly? Out of that bloody mess were coming brown squiggly snakes, and I was horrified that it appeared to be attached to me. It looked like a squished, overly ripe, plump, tomato on my stomach, and, to add to the freak show, skinny garter snakes had risen from the red sludge to feast on the tomato guts.

I started to cry, but my throat seared from the friction of a hard plastic tube that had mysteriously sprouted from my nose and grazed against my throat; I forced myself to cork the flow of tears. I could see fluid flowing from the nasal tube. It wasn't exactly clear, but I couldn't really define the colour. What a monster I had become! How long had this transformation taken? Had I been asleep for hours, days, weeks?

Once the anaesthetic wore off, I became more lucid and learned that while I was asleep during surgery, the doctors had inserted a tube in my nose that went down my throat and into my stomach. This is known as nasogastric (NG) intubation. The purpose of the tube was to drain the contents of my stomach post-surgery. Gastrointestinal secretions and swallowed air (gas) are managed this way while the body recovers. The tube was secured to my nose with tape, a collector bag was placed below my stomach, and gravity continually emptied the contents of my stomach. Sometimes a nurse would suction the tube to ensure everything was being drained.

My head pounded from the repression of tears and all the ghoulish thoughts swirling in my over-stimulated brain. Days later, the doctor said that the post-surgery ostomy bag is transparent to enable the care staff an unobstructed view of my stoma and output, but in regular life my bag would be opaque. The tomato guts were actually my "rosebud," or stoma. I learned that a stoma is a piece of healthy small bowel (the ileum) that has been rerouted from the inside to the outside of the body. The snakes were post-surgery output: some leftover blood in the stool. Talk about ill-prepared. That artiste-nurse must not have seen many roses because the mess on my stomach looked nothing like what I had seen in the garden. It was appalling. The only thing my stoma had in common with a rose was the colour red.

Besides the initial view of my stoma, everything else from those first few days is a blur, except for being allowed to eat half a Popsicle every hour, and watching the pink, orange or red water flow out of my stomach through my NG tube. I'd ask my mum "Please try and get me a pink popsicle, it's the best flavour and I like how it looks coming out of the tube. Orange is my second favourite and red looks like blood." We tried to avoid the cherry flavour, there had been quite enough blood already.

As I was recovering, I met a girl named Linda who also had an ostomy. We were under the same doctor's care and underwent our operations on the same day. "Lin" was fifteen and a feisty teenager, while I had yet to reach puberty, but we connected. Our parents had swapped stories in the surgery waiting rotunda and understood the pain of seeing one's child suffer.

The first few viewings of my belly had a significant enough impact to influence my dreams. Still on regular doses of painkillers, my brain was drugged and full of fear. The sight of my bloody stoma had filled me with dread. The surgery had been a success and I was on a path to recovery, so Dad no longer slept at the hospital, but stayed with me after work until visiting hours were over. As I slept on my first night alone, a nightmare began.

Shit coloured, slimy, slim snakes streamed from my belly en masse and viciously planned to poison the hospital ward. They squiggled out of my stoma, over my stomach, and slid down my legs to the tile floor. Once there, they moved in a pack to find their next victim. The villains' eyes glowed yellow in the dark and it was obvious they were pure evil. I was mute and unable to stop them. The snakes weren't interested in me anyway; I was just the vessel in which they grew. But that couldn't be right, could it? I was not evil, was I? I wanted to get to my new hospital friend, Linda, before the reptiles swarmed, smothered, and killed her. I had to warn her. I had to get to her before they did.

They didn't seem to want to attack me—it was Linda they were after. They were moving fast and multiplying. I couldn't get to her fast enough. I tried.

I tried. I tried. I tried to shout, "Linda, wake up!" but there was no answer. Why couldn't she hear me?

I couldn't stop their growth; soon the hospital floor was teeming with their slithering filth. They crossed the corridor and made their way to Linda. I needed to wake her up. The IV pole would slow me down but I didn't have the nerve to rip it out and attempt to run. I shuffled after the snakes and they looked back at me with their hateful green eyes and taunted me: "too slow, Lindsay, too slow. Keep trying though."

Where were the nurses? Why didn't they see and help me? "Help me, and help Linda. Help!" My lips moved, but no sound came out. The mass of squiggly brown reptiles shuddered in a wave of hateful laughter as they kept moving toward my friend across the hall. They were on a mission and had crossed the threshold of her room. Linda was in the second bed from the door; I still had time. My heart was thumping. Like a cartoon, I could see it pounding through my hospital fatigues. "I can do it," I thought. "I'm stronger than I look. Where are my parents now? Why isn't Linda waking up? The hissing alone should alert her. Is it just me or is everyone else in some sort of fog?"

The snakes were starting to swarm Linda's bed. "HELP." No fucking sound. All I could feel was my cold sweat and terror. Just as the first serpent bore its venomous jaws, I opened my eyes.

I woke up covered in sweat and shaking beside Linda's bed. I could swear my veins were going to pop out of my neck. As my pulse slowed it became clear that I had sleepwalked across the hall to Linda's bed.

The ward was eerie at night. Even when I was awake at night I was usually tucked in my bed and waiting for my next painkiller. It was highly irregular for me to wander around the halls unaccompanied. I clutched my IV pole as I dragged myself back to bed. No nurses saw me, so when I got back to my room, I buzzed them to make sure they hadn't disappeared, and got myself a shot while I had their attention. Bugs, Daffy and Sylvester hadn't been displaced by their unexpected journey. They continued to watch over me from their perch on the pole. The next morning, I told my mum about the dream and sleepwalking, but I didn't tell Linda. Tainting her mind with horrifying thoughts didn't seem like something a friend would do.

—ɯ—

Once my belly had a few days on clear fluids, the NG tube was pulled out of my nose with a forceful tug. Following the initial feeling that my vocal cords were being ripped apart and my stomach pulled out my neck, my throat began to feel normal again. I remained on clear fluids for a day or two. After the Popsicles came Jello, followed by pudding and then once I had handled that, solid food. When real meals went in, they had to come out and that's when I fully understood the function of the bag.

Much to my surprise, it wasn't the size of a garbage bag; it was only 12 inches long. As waste was evacuated from my body via the stoma, it was collected in the bag. I had not been attacked by a blowtorch—the bag was not welded on as I had imagined, but was attached to my body by a waxy flange. The flange was like a sticky baseplate which was taped onto my skin and had a centered, circular Tupperware-like opening that was cut to fit over the stoma. The Tupperware piece of the flange fit together with the connecting Tupperware piece of the bag. Once I realized I had Tupperware and not a Glad Kitchen Catcher, I determined that the bag wasn't as bad as the image I had concocted in my head before surgery.

Dr. Filler, my surgeon, and his residents came by every day on rounds. Everyone had a poke and a look at my new goods. This hardly bothered me anymore as some of them had had their finger up my butt over the last six weeks and had poked and prodded my aching abdomen. Dr. Filler was a kind man and, even though he had sliced me up, I trusted him. Every day he would look at my chart to see my weight and input vs. output. After he spoke with the residents in some medical mumbo jumbo—which I was beginning to understand—he would talk to me directly to find out how I was feeling.

I emptied the contents of my bag into a green plastic measuring cup until the day I left the hospital. When I finally got home, Mum and I pondered how I was going to carry a measuring cup to school with me. No one explained that I would empty my bag into the toilet. Somehow, we figured it out and I got the hang of it.

Chapter 6

The outside

—⚊⚋⚊—

"Sisters function as safety nets in a chaotic world simply by being there for each other."   —Carol Saline

Mum came to get me when I was finally released from the hospital. I was ensconced in a wheelchair wearing a pink tracksuit, my purple padded coat, and a black wool scarf and hat. As I was being wheeled out of my room, I gave my *Looney Tunes* IV decorations to a younger girl in my room who had admired them. Bugs and his pals could comfort someone else now.

As we left the ward, Mum and I made a pit stop to say goodbye to Linda—she was leaving the next day. Lin and I held hands as we said goodbye and she said, "Make sure you keep in touch."

"I will," I said, "You too. I hope you get to go home tomorrow." Our mothers exchanged phone numbers and we used them. Thus began a friendship that endures until this day.

Mum and I exited, leaving a trail of commotion in our wake. There were many nurses to wish me well and ask that we come back and see them when I was feeling fit and strong. With all the fuss created, I felt like a bit of a celebrity. On our elevator ride down to street level, I imagined that I received pitying stares so I shrank in my seat, in a vain attempt to hide. Then the doors opened and I could taste freedom. When we reached the EXIT sign, a stream of light was coming through the sliding glass doors. I had to squint.

We were just outside the gift shop, and I asked Mum, "Can you help me out of this chair so I can sit on over there and wait?"

Out of the confines of the chair, I felt one step closer to "normal." Once I was safely perched on the bench, Mum dashed to retrieve the car. It was mid-day and quiet. No sirens, no moans, no TV, no beeping IV poles. I was left to enjoy a few peaceful moments in the hospital entryway.

As I was taking in the sights, a man with a professional-looking camera came up to me and asked whether he could take my photo for a hospital pamphlet of some sort. I had been told over and over again not to talk to strangers, but this guy only wanted a photo and there were several orderlies taking a break nearby, so I said OK. It was nice being seen by someone in a positive way. Everything in hospital had felt so ugly, including me, so being a "model" for a moment was a temptation I couldn't resist.

The photographer snapped a few shots of me looking at a painting on the wall and then asked me for my address so he could send me a copy of the photo. I was a scaredy-cat by nature and quietly explained that he would have to wait for my mum. He understood and asked me a few questions about why I had been in hospital.

The reality of the situation set in. This wasn't a fashion shoot. I wasn't a model. I was still a patient and if I needed to escape, I was too weak to do so. My heart began to beat fast in fear as I talked to him, because I wondered if this seemingly nice guy was actually a "bad man" and I had been naive in thinking him harmless. As I began to sweat, Mum appeared and, judging by the worry on her face, the man thought it prudent to promptly give her a business card and account for his presence by explaining the significance of the painting on the wall behind me, and why he had photographed me admiring the artwork.

That was enough for Mum—she gave him our address, and he wished us well, promising to send a photo. True to his word, an 8 × 10, black and white, side profile shot of me arrived in the mail several weeks later. By then, I was feeling less weak and I could enjoy the fact that I had been a "model" even if it was in the context of being a sick kid.

As the photographer left, I turned around and looked out the automatic sliding doors again. Parked outside was Mum's gleaming black sedan. The sun was reflecting off the car's surface in a dazzling effect. It looked like the car was covered in crystals. This gem of a car was going to take me home. It was a few days before Halloween and the air slipping in through the front doors was crisp. I gingerly placed myself on the front passenger leather seat and breathed in the familiar smell of this well-kept car. My nose had missed the scents of leather and Armor All. For almost two months my senses had been robbed of many pleasures. They had been inundated with cold metal, antiseptic, blood and poop. The comfort of leather was astounding; how had I not noticed this before?

As we drove away from the hospital, I felt a disconcerting mixture of joy and fear. I think I know what prisoners feel like when they finally experience the Outside again. You leave behind the safety of your cell and routine. On the Outside, you are responsible for your new life. No more shots of Demerol for pain, no more doctors to assure you that all the different aches and pains are normal, no more security blanket buzzer for the nurse (I rarely used the buzzer, but it was nice to know it was there). What would life be like at home with my new appendage? How would I empty my bag at school? Would my sister Courtenay still love me? These thoughts ran through my head but dissipated when I began to focus on the sights of the city. Downtown Toronto looked astoundingly colourful; the grass, leaves and buildings were so bright; had everything just been freshly painted? From the Inside, when I had glimpsed out of the windows, things hadn't seemed so alive.

As we rolled into our neighbourhood, I noticed how many trees and well-groomed gardens there were. We rounded a corner to our street, and I imagined I was in a Disney movie. The street was lined with trees, and with the autumn foliage out in full force it resembled the entranceway to the castle in *Beauty and the Beast*. I rolled down my window and sucked in the smell. Birds were chirping, and squirrels were looking for food in the early afternoon October sun. Maybe

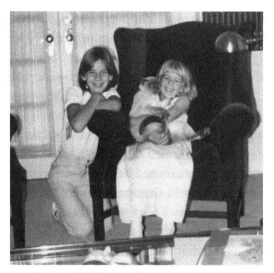

Me, Courtenay, and Suki at home, right before I got sick. August, 1980.

I wanted to do something special for Court. Dad had given me a box filled with loose change he'd saved for many months. We counted and rolled the coins so he could take them to the bank, and he gave me the cash. It was just under 100 dollars. I had Mum drive me down to Yonge Street and went into the card shop—it had the best stuffed animals. Courtenay was allergic to Suki, so couldn't cuddle with her. I bought the biggest, prettiest stuffed kitty in the store. It was white and fluffy with blue eyes and a pink satin bow. It cost more than a third of my money. I saved the rest for later and went home to present my sister with a cat that wouldn't make her wheeze.

As the photographer left, I turned around and looked out the automatic sliding doors again. Parked outside was Mum's gleaming black sedan. The sun was reflecting off the car's surface in a dazzling effect. It looked like the car was covered in crystals. This gem of a car was going to take me home. It was a few days before Halloween and the air slipping in through the front doors was crisp. I gingerly placed myself on the front passenger leather seat and breathed in the familiar smell of this well-kept car. My nose had missed the scents of leather and Armor All. For almost two months my senses had been robbed of many pleasures. They had been inundated with cold metal, antiseptic, blood and poop. The comfort of leather was astounding; how had I not noticed this before?

As we drove away from the hospital, I felt a disconcerting mixture of joy and fear. I think I know what prisoners feel like when they finally experience the Outside again. You leave behind the safety of your cell and routine. On the Outside, you are responsible for your new life. No more shots of Demerol for pain, no more doctors to assure you that all the different aches and pains are normal, no more security blanket buzzer for the nurse (I rarely used the buzzer, but it was nice to know it was there). What would life be like at home with my new appendage? How would I empty my bag at school? Would my sister Courtenay still love me? These thoughts ran through my head but dissipated when I began to focus on the sights of the city. Downtown Toronto looked astoundingly colourful; the grass, leaves and buildings were so bright; had everything just been freshly painted? From the Inside, when I had glimpsed out of the windows, things hadn't seemed so alive.

As we rolled into our neighbourhood, I noticed how many trees and well-groomed gardens there were. We rounded a corner to our street, and I imagined I was in a Disney movie. The street was lined with trees, and with the autumn foliage out in full force it resembled the entranceway to the castle in *Beauty and the Beast*. I rolled down my window and sucked in the smell. Birds were chirping, and squirrels were looking for food in the early afternoon October sun. Maybe it was that other Disney classic *Snow White* that I was in, because I envisioned the birds painting make-believe hearts above my head. Why had I not realized before that my home was like a castle? From near death to Disney, perspective became a powerful resource from that moment on.

I thought if someone could take a photo of me at this moment, I would appear on the film as a flash of light, because my insides felt so full of gladness. My outside was still tender, but surely this light that I was full of and surrounded by would quickly heal me. I said to my mum, "Everything looks so vivid and wonderful . . . it's amazing." The effect was dazzling. We went inside our house and I thought not only was my house bright, it was cozy and warm. Most importantly, the space was mine.

I wanted to see my bedroom, on the third floor with Courtenay's. She was at school so the house was quiet. We climbed the stairs slowly calling out to Suki, our Siamese cat, as we made our ascent. Suki had been sleeping in the sunshine on Mum and Dad's bed, but she didn't need much coaxing to follow us.

At the top of the stairs, on the left-hand side, was my bedroom. I had chosen to decorate it in yellow, my favourite colour. Yellow floral wallpaper, yellow bedding and a white carpet made for a very cheery setting, which was just what the doctor ordered. My shelves were lined with framed family photos, and Aunt Jill had added a recent one of Su and me that had been taken at JC Penney's that summer. We both had big smiles, sparkly, happy eyes and emanated health with our summer tans. Courtenay and I shared a closet—I checked in on my clothes and was not surprised that everything seemed in order. After the hike to the third floor and all the excitement of being home, I needed a nap. Mum brought me some banana bread and chocolate milk (it was time to fatten me up!) and I slept with Suki in the crook of my arm for several hours. Her even purr and velvety fur had a hypnotic effect. My reality was now warm and fuzzy, compared to the harsh climate I had just left. I savoured every moment.

I woke up to Court standing over me, deep breathing in that allergy-ridden way she had. She snored like an old man, but looked like an angel.

My sister was a beautiful, blonde, outgoing ray of six-year-old sunshine. She exclaimed, "You're back!" and hugged me. She was clearly happy to have her big sister home.

I suddenly realized how much I had needed to see her. Courtenay had spent the last seven weeks being farmed out to babysitters and friends' houses. Hospital regulations prevented her from visiting me while I had been "away"—when you are in Grade 1 you were labelled as a walking germ and too big a health risk for the patients. Dad had tried unsuccessfully to sneak her in to visit me once, but apart from that she had no real concept as to what had been happening to me and why I had taken Mum and Dad with me, except that I was sick. What she was aware of was that this new "bag" I had been given garnered much attention and that maybe she would like one too.

A few days after I arrived home, I was changing my appliance when Court joined me in the bathroom in her underwear. She had a white sports sock tucked in her Smurfs panties, and while placing her pudgy hands on her hips and pushing her belly out she piped, "Look Lins, I have a bag too!"

I could play this game. "Are you sure you want a bag?" I probed.

"Yep, but I don't have any flange or tape like you," she said.

Well, we fixed that up right away by taking some of my excess flange and carefully pasting it below her belly button. Then we added some of my waterproof tape and she was all set. Courtenay had a sock-bag and was quite pleased with herself. This game grew old within a few weeks but it served its purpose in helping me to understand Court's feelings. She had been isolated from a major family event. Her big sister had been sick, deserted her, and hogged all of Mum and Dad's energy and time for what probably seemed like years in kid time. We needed to bond. She and I had trundle beds and took turns sleeping together in each other's rooms for several months after I returned from hospital. We needed to be close to each other.

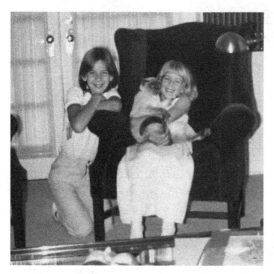

Me, Courtenay, and Suki at home, right before I got sick. August, 1980.

I wanted to do something special for Court. Dad had given me a box filled with loose change he'd saved for many months. We counted and rolled the coins so he could take them to the bank, and he gave me the cash. It was just under 100 dollars. I had Mum drive me down to Yonge Street and went into the card shop—it had the best stuffed animals. Courtenay was allergic to Suki, so couldn't cuddle with her. I bought the biggest, prettiest stuffed kitty in the store. It was white and fluffy with blue eyes and a pink satin bow. It cost more than a third of my money. I saved the rest for later and went home to present my sister with a cat that wouldn't make her wheeze.

Chapter 7

Back to school

—ᴍ—

"'Tis the last rose of summer, left blooming all alone; all her lovely companions are faded and gone." —Thomas Moore

My Grade 6 teacher, Mrs. Grant, had paid me a visit a couple of weeks after I had been admitted to hospital. She brought me the last rose from her garden and sat by my bed, stroking my hair while I dozed on and off. She was a gentle lady, with short, auburn hair and a kind smile. She explained that because it was late in the season, and the rose was in full bloom, it signified strength. I liked that and thought the rose continued to be pretty even as the pink petals began to drop off. Unfortunately, a few weeks later, my "rosebud" stoma had me angrily telling my mum, "The nurse said it would look like a rose! It's not pretty, it's gross!" As an adult, I never buy red roses, sticking to pink, white or yellow.

As I regained strength after the first surgery, I was eager to get back to a regular routine. I returned to my Grade 6 classroom for half days. Most of my contemporaries were kind and I was welcomed back with a huge banner across an entire wall of the classroom. It was really cool because it was a computer print out; this was new technology, and I recently learned that Richard, a boy in my class, had his father do it for me. I can just imagine the size and noise of the machinery needed then to produce such a big banner. This was cutting edge stuff and I was impressed!

Not everyone was so thoughtful. In my first hour back, a girl in my class, who had always walked with her nose in the air, interrogated me. "Why is your hair so thin?" she asked loudly.

The question felt like an attack. I managed to explain that the anesthetic made a lot of my hair fall out, but that it would grow back. I was calm on the outside but scared shitless on the inside. Would everyone be this insensitive? Was I going to be the class freak? Mrs. Grant had explained to my peers while I had been gone what was happening, but probably most of them didn't really comprehend her explanation. Still, she did her best to prepare the class for my return, and I'm sure it helped. My parents agreed with Mrs. Grant that explaining my surgery to the Grade 6 students would assist in demystifying the situation. She was like a goalie, catching many of the hard questions for me. Some were bound to slip through though.

Many of my classmates had sent me get-well cards while I had been in hospital, particularly my best friend, Jane, who handmade some very fun, imaginative cards that always made me smile. Some other people also came to visit me while I was in the slammer. Marcus, a boy who had a crush on me at the time, plucked up the nerve to come and see me, accompanied by his friend, Reg. Mum and Cindy the nurse gussied me up as best they could before they let Marcus and Reg in. Mum slathered my lips with Chapstick, combed my bed head, straightened the bedding, and made sure I was decent (my butt and non-existent boobs covered). However, the moon face from the prednisone and several tubes linking me to various pieces of equipment were all too much for Reg who, after taking a quick peek, disappeared out the door and down the hall. Marcus smiled, came to my bedside and had a visit that was short (the best kind) but obviously meaningful, as I remember it to this day. I was all nerves, and excited that a boy had made the trip to see me. Marcus and I recently connected on Facebook and I thanked him for his visit when I was sick. We ended up having an exchange that was meaningful for both of us.

As the springy pink hand had promised, about two weeks after Halloween my new Calvin Klein jeans and Little Heroes arrived from Los Angeles. Four pairs of new jeans and three different colours of the Indian cotton track suits. Aunt Jill had pinned a different brooch on each top. There was a rainbow, butterfly, and flamingo. My chin length, brown hair was thin, but my beanpole body looked fashionable in my new duds. Mum and Aunt Jill had taught me the art of shopping from an early age. Aunt Jill had unlimited resources, but my mum knew how to get the most bang for her buck. She was definitely one of the most stylish mums in our neighbourhood. She still is. Both women taught me my love of clothes and the importance of looking good when you feel bad. They told me that when you look like you are taking care of yourself, people aren't scared to be around you and treat you like you are healthy. Furthermore, maintaining a feeling of normalcy is helpful to you and those who love you, although, throughout the years, I have had many moments where I thought "to hell with it" and allowed myself to look as bad as I felt. Sometimes it's good for people to understand that you are having a bad day.

Upon my return to school, no one asked me about my ileostomy, which recently made me wonder if that part of the story was left out. The other day I asked Jane and she confirmed that Mrs. Grant just spoke about the surgery, not my bag. It was hidden underneath my clothes so no one knew about it unless I told them. I liked it being invisible. I was embarrassed by its function and worried about people thinking I was dirty. I only told my three closest girlfriends about my bag. The spring of Grade 6, my class took a four-day overnight trip to Boyne River and I was given special permission to use the teacher's bathroom instead of the student dorm showers and toilets. I was uncomfortable being singled out, but that was the price I had to pay for keeping my privacy.

The school excursion was how I imagined camp must be. There was a nondescript, dank, girls' dormitory where we slept in bunk beds, and when we went to the cafeteria we sang "Johnny Appleseed" before tucking in to breakfast. There was another group of kids at Boyne River while we were there. It was a Grade 6 class from an inner-city school in Toronto, and we shared the bus drive to the rustic river retreat with them. There was one bus for the girls and a different one for the boys.

The day before we left on our adventure, Mrs. Grant had encouraged us to branch out and try to meet the kids from the other school. When the bus arrived, it was already half full with the girls from the downtown school; they looked older than us. As we boarded, I noticed that most of my crowd seemed very unsure of our bus mates. Neither group acknowledged each other, but, instead of just ignoring the strangers, a few of our girls seemed to snicker out the side of their mouths, and others seemed genuinely nervous. I was embarrassed by their behaviour. Just because our shirts had little alligators and polo players embroidered on the chest didn't make us better than anyone else. My experience in hospital had made that very clear. To me, our left-over tans from March break were a display of good fortune, not superiority. Also, our healthy glows were more noticeable because we were all white, the other group was more diverse.

I had shared hospital rooms with people from all areas of the city, of different races and religions, and we all had our own stories. My mum and dad hadn't thought twice about assisting other girls when their parents weren't able to be with them. It was during my first stay in hospital that I noticed not everyone was as well dressed as my parents and that, in general, we seemed more affluent than many of the people sharing my ward. Pre-colitis I had been aware that not everyone lived as well as we did, but I had been relatively sheltered from the less fortunate areas of the city. Visiting Vermont each summer didn't exactly broaden my socioeconomic scope, except I learned how the really rich lived. The Hospital for Sick Children is located in downtown Toronto, and it was while I was there that I began to understand how few people lived lives like ours. Trips to Florida, horseback riding, big backyards and nice cars were far from average, and I became very thankful that Mum didn't have to work and could stay at my bedside. It would have been a completely different experience if I had been alone in the hospital during the day and evenings. I had my mum and dad to be my voice with the nurses and doctors; many people didn't have that luxury.

What I know now is, everybody suffers. Some people endure their pain privately, others share their woes. What one person considers

Chapter 8

Sitz down

—◠◡◠—

"Shame derives its power from being unspeakable." —Brené Brown

By Grade 7, I had grown out of my Calvin Kleins and was starting junior high school. The doctors had advised me that my ostomy could be temporary, and once I felt strong enough, we could have two operations to put me back to "normal." When I say "we," I am referring to the fact that although my parents' stomachs weren't being sliced open, their hearts were each time I was operated on. They might as well have been on the table with me. Mum and Dad have each said to me separately that if they could have had the operations and pain for me, they would have. Even if that were possible, I wouldn't give my ill health to either one of them. It was my journey to muck my way through.

My experience with illness was horrendous. I wouldn't wish it on my worst enemy. However, every now and then, I used to daydream that it would be very satisfying to transfer my overactive autoimmune system to a heinous murderer or child abuser. Just as women will discuss transferring the fat from their butt to their boobs, or donating their excess pounds to a skinny friend, I have imagined scooping up my diseases and hurling them at a criminal rotting away in a cell. I figured they deserved more suffering, so they could take mine. This wasn't a common fantasy for me, but it did cross my mind from time to time.

I had the first of two "hook-up" surgeries during the week of my Grade 7 March Break. In this operation, my bowels were prepared for Operation #2 when my ileum (part of my small intestine) would be reconnected to my anus and I would be able to poop normally again. My sphincter muscles had deteriorated over 18 months of disuse. After Operation #1 of the hook-up surgeries, my bag remained, and my butt was prepped for use and leaked small amounts.

I had a tough time controlling myself but had to get my muscles into action again. I wore sanitary pads to catch any poo drainage that I couldn't control. This resulted in a sort of diaper rash that I tried to alleviate by taking colloidal oatmeal sitz baths. The rash got so bad that, at one point, I was doing the sitz baths in the school nurse's bathroom at lunchtime. I would try and slide into the office when the hallways weren't busy so people didn't notice where I was going. I wanted to be under the radar, invisible.

I shared the space with an outspoken, tough, red-headed girl named Moira, who was doing her kidney dialysis treatments. Moira sat on the window sill hooked up to her machine, and I sat in the bathroom with the door open so we could chat. Moira revealed her life in clipped ways:

"My dad left us when I was young."

"Mom gets home late from her job so I have a key to let myself in."

"I've lost count how many times I've been in hospital."

It was again clear to me that although my situation wasn't easy, it could have been much harder. I tried to down play some of the facts of my life and the one-time Moira forgot her house key and I invited her over after school until her mum was home, I felt guilty about my big, well decorated house. I could hear her thinking, "Must be nice."

This vulnerable seating situation of our lunch times reminded me of when I first got my bag, how, at my request, Su would take pictures of me on the toilet (with my bag and privates covered) because I wanted to prove that I was "normal." Until I started writing this book, it didn't occur to me how different I must have felt to consider what amounts to a bathroom selfie as being normal.

On the outside I was coping very well, but years later I realized how much shame I felt about my bag. I wasn't aware then of the fear, anger and sadness inside of me. It was too much to contemplate. My mind was very busy coping with my health in the moment and the day-to-day life of a teenager. That was hard enough, I don't think my brain was ready to delve into more trauma, I just wanted to belong like everybody else. I recognized that Moira's hard exterior was a defence and I understood why, but I didn't want to be like that.

Only Moira and my two best friends were aware of what was going on or where I was at lunch. No one else knew. No one teased me and my invisibility endured. It was the only way I knew how to get through things at the time.

Chapter 9

Hooked up

—✳︎—

"A mother's arms are more comforting than anyone else." —Princess Diana

The second of the two hook-up operations was planned for four months later, the summer before Grade 8. We didn't want me to miss school, so we tried to take advantage of any holiday time for surgery and recovery. That summer ended up being the worst of my life.

Summertime for me was equated with Vermont; carefree days, outside and active. Sunshine and scary surgeries felt incongruous. Most of the summers I'd spent in Vermont were some of the best of my life. Still, during my teens, I frequently joked with Mum, saying "Vermont is my bad luck spot." When I was about nine, my cousin, Jason, had been swinging me on the tire swing; I was squealing with joy until I inadvertently crashed, head first, into the tree. Uncle Charlie gave me a cold raw steak to soothe the swelling of my black eye, but Jason felt so badly, that it was me who consoled him. That winter in Vermont I collided with a different tree while tobogganing with my cousins. Mum gave me pack of frozen peas to reduce my swelling eye that time. The next summer, I came down with a raging case of impetigo on my buttocks—I had peed in some poison ivy—and it took weeks of sitz baths to clear it up. I hadn't realized it at the time, but my first symptoms of ulcerative colitis started in Vermont and two winters after I had my ostomy surgery, I broke my wrist skiing at our favourite ski hill in Vermont.

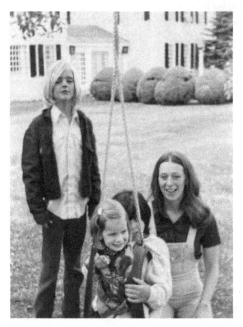

Val, Jason, me, and Mum at the tire swing. Summer, 1973.

Looking back on it, we were incredibly active in Vermont. Accidents were inevitable; I'm surprised there weren't more of them, and more serious ones. Su and I were outside all day. We were on horses bareback, with no helmet or reins and thought nothing of it. We would ride in the back of the pick-up truck bouncing around with the dogs. Su's trampoline was big, but it had no net walls to protect us. We'd fearlessly fly around on that thing and never got hurt. Climbing trees was a pastime and in the winter, we'd slide around near the *mostly* frozen pond on our sleds. From my perspective now, maybe Vermont was my "good luck spot." Regardless, in Grade 8, I didn't believe in bad luck so I was looking forward to getting to Vermont after I recovered from my operation that was scheduled for late June.

The doctors had assured us that I had the best chance they had ever seen of a successful hook-up surgery, so we were full of expectations for my return to a bag-free existence. When I was sent home following Operation #2 my family had a "bag burning" ceremony on the steps of our back patio. The garden was in full bloom and looked suitably festive for our celebration. Surrounded by tall cedar hedges, bright pink peonies, pink and white rose bushes, Japanese maple trees, as well as other lush plants and bushes, I placed a bag, flange and tape in an aluminum foil pan and Dad lit the match as I said "Adios, ostomy! Bye bye to my bag!"

We were optimistic despite the fact that I was failing to put on any weight and it was too early to establish how successful the surgery had been. My output was so difficult to control that I had been subconsciously compensating by reducing my input. After about two weeks at home and daily doses of pain medication, Metamucil, Imodium and Ensure, things were not improving.

To be closer to my parents, sister, and reduce my stairs, I was sleeping in the second-floor guest room with Courtenay. I tried not to look in the mirror when I visited the bathroom. When I finally snuck a peek at myself, it felt like a dream sequence in a movie . . .

I squinted and tried to focus. I recognized that girl. She looked so different, but I knew her. . . I asked myself, why was she so gaunt? Also, I thought she had altered the way she wore her hair—it had been thinned. Since when did she wear track pants in the middle of the day? She used to be one of the best-dressed kids around. My friend . . . she was coming into focus . . . my friend had lost her sparkle; she looked emaciated and defeated. As I got closer, I saw that her eyes were hollowed. The mirror was reflecting a crystal-clear image now. I no longer needed to squint. I was flooded by a wave of nausea. She was me.

It was shocking. Where did I go? It was all too clear that this had not been a nightmare; this was real. I saw the prescription pain medication with my name on it on the bathroom counter, and an image of me swallowing the entire bottle of small blue pills crystallized in my brain. I picked up the potent little candies, released the lid, and suddenly lost control of my hand. It was as if someone had flipped a vibrate switch at my right elbow and, with that, the pills spilled all over the cold tile floor. Through my tears I gathered what I could find of the Demerol and sat on the toilet holding my head in my hands, staring at the white porcelain floor until the trembling in my body ceased.

I can't remember how long I sat until I felt that my legs would take me safely back to bed. As I disappeared underneath the covers, I resolved that I didn't need to consult a mirror again for a long while. I felt like someone should have warned me, but what would my mum have said? "Be careful of the mirrors. . . they might bite you in the ass," or "My sweet baby, you look a step away from death, please avoid the looking glass." It was through therapy that this memory was revisited and I was allowed to weep for the little girl in the movie in my brain. I think back to that time, and still have to remind myself that that poor, straggly little pip was me. I want to wrap her in my arms and tell her life won't always be this hard, that she will thrive again, and that her small weak body harbours an enormous spirit.

—ɯ—

Age thirteen, I weighed sixty-three pounds, and had noticed that my urine was tinged with stool. My mother phoned the hospital and was convinced by whoever was on the other end of the phone that this was impossible and I must have been sitting at a "funny angle" on the toilet. By now, I was finely tuned to my body's idiosyncrasies and knew that I was not hallucinating, but it seemed I required cold hard evidence. I got my proof soon enough.

Intense stomach cramps sent me back to the hospital and, although I strongly protested, a nurse inserted a tampon to test my story. Bingo. My last surgery had left a tiny hole in my rectal wall. They had to go in and patch the leak. More surgery, more IV's, another catheter, another NG tube and another round of Demerol shots. At thirteen, I was getting to be an old pro.

This time I didn't make it home because it was obvious to all involved that my body was not taking well to being reconnected. I was in agony and, according to my nurse, was being injected intravenously with enough morphine to "put out a horse" with no relief. I didn't want to be a nuisance but couldn't stop moaning in pain. I was in a shared room and I felt bad for my roommate and my parents, but I couldn't stifle my groans, the pain was too intense. I writhed in bed, trying to find a comfortable position. I was beside myself with misery. Dr. Filler didn't let me suffer too long. While Mum was in the hallway calling Dad, I asked a nurse to take me to the bathroom and, when I was dragging myself back to bed, I saw Mum sobbing at the end of the corridor. She was a crumpled ball on the sofa and Dr. Filler had his hand resting on her shoulder and was speaking in hushed tones. I knew what was next and felt some relief that the pain might soon be over.

Dr. Filler came by my bed and explained that the next morning I would be having another surgery to re-attach my stoma. At that moment, I wondered if I might die before the morning, and the bag seemed like a blessing, because it had provided me health.

I suffered through the night, and was prepped an hour earlier than planned for the morning surgery. They wanted to wheel me down but Mum hadn't arrived at the hospital yet. There was no way I was going to be taken away alone, without my mummy or daddy. They called home and Mum sped down University Avenue while Dad made arrangements for Courtenay.

This time, they took me to wait outside the operating room and made my parents stay in the waiting area. I was able to watch the doctors come and go down the long empty corridor. It was very quiet. I saw Dr. Filler through a glass window, in an office of some sort. He was still in his civilian clothes, and was eating a sandwich. Something so mundane and necessary, but I was infuriated. Couldn't they at least put me out while the team was getting nourished? Why did I have to wait alone while my doctor enjoyed his breakfast? As he walked by, I angrily questioned him, "How much longer?"

It was obvious by his expression that he hadn't expected to see me waiting in the hall, and was surprised by my tone. He simply replied, "Soon Lindsay, soon."

When I woke up from the surgery the surprise element was gone; I knew what I was in for during the recovery period. Aunt Jill came to Toronto again to visit during my hospital stay and didn't leave until the day before I went home. When I first saw her, she gave me several hardcover books about Princess Diana. Like most of the world, I was captivated by Lady Di and couldn't get enough of her "fairy tale" story. Leafing through those books, which were mostly photos, provided a great distraction. Mum, my aunt, and I loved talking about Diana's clothes and jewelry. During that time, if I had to choose between a *Majesty* or *Seventeen* magazine, *Majesty* would win if the princess was on the cover. Aunt Jill also brought a bag of wrapped gifts to the hospital and left them on my bedside table so that I could open one each morning when I woke up alone. I found all sorts of treasures inside, including novels, games, a kaleidoscope and a gold necklace with a pendant of a carved wooden horse's head. She had bought all the goodies in Woodstock, Vermont at The Unicorn, my favourite store. Mum took the necklace home for safe keeping; I still wear it sometimes. The kaleidoscope brightened my drab hospital world with its swirls of colour, especially after a dose of Demerol. It was like I was in a psychedelic music video: funky and fun.

The doctors had made the decision to spare me an NG tube when they performed the surgery to give me back my bag. I had been through a miserable month and we were all disappointed that the two hook-up surgeries had not been successful. The hope was that I wouldn't need the uncomfortable nose tube and I would pass my intestinal fluids at a safe rate on my own. That didn't happen. Aunt Jill was at my bedside when Dr. Filler came by to tell me that I needed an NG tube for my recovery. He apologized to me that they hadn't inserted one when I was under anaesthesia. He had been hoping I could get by without the drainage tube to spare me the discomfort. The intention was good and I could tell he felt genuinely sorry. We were informed that someone was coming by shortly to insert a tube. This would happen while I was awake.

Aunt Jill turned pale. She and Dad don't have strong stomachs for medical procedures. When I broke my wrist skiing in Vermont. My aunt, dad and mum rushed me to hospital, but Dad and Aunt Jill went a shade of pale green when the doctor explained how they would reset the bone without anaesthesia. They left the room to get some cold air, while Mum held my hand through the quick but agonizing procedure. I didn't need the benefit of that future experience, or to see her pallor, to know that my aunt was uncomfortable. I assured her that she didn't need to stay and watch, or hold my hand. I was confident that Mum would be back in time to be there for me. Poor Mum, she did return to watch them try with three different sized tubes before they got the right fit. I gagged as I was directed to swallow to help the tube go down. Aunt Jill could hear me choking on the other side of the curtain and she crept out of the room. I squeezed my mum's hand like my life depended on it. Her hand felt like my lifeline.

Chapter 10

Truth or dare

—ɯ—

*"The real truth, that dare not speak itself, is that no one is in control.
Absolutely no one."* —Terence McKenna

A month later, in mid-August, I was well enough to make a trip to Vermont. This year it would be different. There was a new member in our family, Katrina. Katrina's mother had died in the spring and left her alone. Aunt Jill had been a friend of Katrina's mother, and took in Katrina and her dog Bobo as members of the Bronson family. I had written a letter to Katrina in the spring and sent her some colourful stickers. She was one year older than me and had been through the most traumatic episode of her life. She and her mum had been sleeping together when her mother had a heart attack in the middle of the night. Her mother died in her arms, while Katrina screamed for help. This 14-year-old girl, with no siblings and a father who was almost non-existent in her life, suddenly had to assimilate into the Bronson clan. I wanted to make her feel welcome because I couldn't imagine the horror of what had happened to her, and how alone she must have felt. I understood the world could play mean tricks on you, but I always got better from my times of sickness; her mother wasn't coming back.

Vermont was different this year too because Aunt Jill had invited Su's friend Libby to the farm for the time that I would be there, and because Mum, Dad and Court were joining me for part of the trip. The dynamics were vastly different from previous years and, as empathetic as I was to Katrina, I felt I had been replaced as Su's surrogate sister. Now she had a big sister for real. Libby was along to make sure we were a foursome, instead of a potentially problematic threesome. I guess no one considered Court in this equation, but she was only there for six days with Mum and Dad. Her severe allergy to horses made Vermont an uncomfortable place to be.

Aunt Jill bought Katrina, Su and me coordinating jean skirts and vests; we looked like a gangly version of the Spice Girls. I liked Katrina and Libby, they were fun, but a nasty feeling of being a commodity surfaced again as I felt I had been so easily replaced in Su's life. If I wasn't a playmate for Su, then I just became a friend for Katrina. I felt I had no choice in what my role was supposed to be.

It's hard to see things clearly when you're a teenager, and under-neath all the girlish fun we had that year, I felt confused. Su was an important part of my life, and I wasn't used to sharing her. I wanted Katrina to feel welcome, and when jealousy crept into my conscious-ness, it was quickly intermingled with guilt. This girl had just lost her mother. I should not feel envy.

Katrina and I got along well, and I understood when she felt left out. Over the years, I too had experienced the insecurity that family dynamics sometimes fostered. She and I took many long walks dur-ing that first summer. We discussed her mum, her new family, and how to cope with and understand the uncertainties of life. In later years, I talked about that summer with Su and Katrina separately. I learned that Su also felt the situation bewildering at times. I had been her only summer companion, and I was now forging a relation-ship with her new sister too. I think none of us really knew where we fit in, but we all wanted it to work.

—⁂—

That summer, I was alone in our bedroom when Aunt Jill popped her head in. "Lindsay-loo, do you want to go with me to Woodstock? I'll take you shopping. Charlie is going to stay here with the others, so it can just be you and me. I think it's time you have some pretty under things." Then, she grinned and gave me a saucy wink.

I was curious about why I was getting this special treatment, and felt very excited about having alone time with my aunt. That was rare. It felt like a gift. I didn't care what we were buying and quickly answered, "That sounds fun, I'll just get changed."

On the car ride to town, Aunt Jill brought me up to date on what was going on with the family in England and asked me if I had any crushes on boys at school. I did, but I didn't think about them much during the summer months.

After we parked, Aunt Jill led me to an exclusive lingerie store tucked in a corner of town. I had never been inside. The way the staff fawned over my aunt, it was clear she was a regular customer— "Mrs. Bronson, so good to see you again!" they said, over and over.

Aunt Jill explained that she was there with me, her niece, and she wanted to buy me some lacy bodysuits for when I started dating. She explained that men were very visual and that camouflaging my bag with pretty lingerie would make me more alluring. That sounded reasonable, so I took her word for it. I loved being around the satin and lace, and we had fun as I tried on lots of sexy underwear. "Ooooh, look at you in THAT!" she'd say, or "I think the red is too tarty, let's try it in blush . . ."

I hadn't come close to being naked with boys yet but, as I vamped in the change room, I loved being treated like an adult and looking like one too. My aunt had often made me feel pretty, she did my hair when we were going out, and bought me fashionable clothes. Su was a bit of a tomboy so her mom enjoyed being girly with me. Now, she was trying to make me feel comfortable with my sexuality. She asked the sales girl, "She has such a good figure, doesn't she?" My aunt was beautiful, so I loved her seeing me as feminine and attractive. It was an intoxicating feeling having her undivided attention, being fussed over and viewed as a lovely young woman, instead of a sick teenager.

We left the store with a bag full of goodies carefully wrapped in pale pink tissue paper. She bought me something white, pink, nude and black, a carefully chosen assortment of colours. For years, those teddies stayed folded in my underwear drawer. Just looking at them made me feel feminine. They also reminded me of my aunt's love for me, as well as her good, but misguided intentions. She didn't mean to inflict damage on my self-esteem, but she had forgotten that young boys just want in your knickers, they don't care if they are lacy or not. I didn't need to hide my bag behind lace. I needed to love my body. I needed to know that my ileostomy didn't make me less appealing.

—⚋—

That summer, Aunt Jill and Uncle Charlie had planned a special excursion to New York City for all of us. We spent four exciting days in the Big Apple seeing a Broadway show each day, and dining at celebrated restaurants every afternoon or evening. It was during this time that Su, Katrina and I got our kicks playing Truth or Dare, and we made it our mission to get everyone involved in the hilarities. Dad was particularly game this trip and accepted each dare with abandon. Uncle Charlie opted out of the games and we went easy on our demands of Mum and Aunt Jill. One evening, we dared my dad to dance around Windows of the World, the restaurant at the top of the World Trade Center, with a rose clenched between his teeth. He glided around four neighbouring tables doing just as we requested and, as he sat back down to dinner, a fellow diner approached him for his autograph. She was convinced he was an actor and had enjoyed his display of joie de vivre. I never quite knew whether this amused Uncle Charlie as he sat there as one of the biggest box office draws of the time. I like to think he enjoyed the irony.

The next night, Su was quiet at dinner for a while before piping up, "Uncle John, I double-dare you to moon out the back of the window of your limo!"

After the girls' giggling subsided, my father raised his eyebrow, and did a half bow as he replied, "I accept your dare, my dear; you'd better keep your eyes peeled on the drive home."

Mum and Aunt Jill exclaimed, "John!" in unison, although in slightly different tones. Mum might have been uncertain and Aunt Jill seemed delighted.

Two cars had been driving us around for our NYC stay. There was one for the adults and one for the five girls. Uncle Charlie had been sitting up front in their limo and he was decidedly uncomfortable with

Dad accepting Su's dare. I think that night he sorely regretted opting out of the tinted window option. Aunt Jill and my mother were egging Dad on; this was just the type of mischief that Aunt Jill loved. As my father was preparing to pull his pants down, our car was directly behind the adults and we were leaning on top of each other into the front seat to prepare for a good view. Dad didn't disappoint us. His bare white ass was clearly visible out the back window of their Lincoln and we fell back into our seats doubled over in gleeful giggles. The Bronsons' secretary, Sue, who doubled as our chaperone, ended up with the best view as she rode in the front of our car. She shared in the hilarity as we returned to the hotel after our successful evening of dinner and dares.

It was years later that I discovered that Uncle Charlie had planned and paid for that trip to New York because Dad had been diagnosed with an arteriovenous malformation (AVM) in his brain, and his neurologist had advised him "to get his affairs in order." My parents had just seen me through hell, and then Dad, unbeknownst to Court and me, had gone to a neurologist because of earaches. As well as a benign tumour in his ear, the CAT scan revealed a malformed vein in his brain. Mum and Dad had been led to believe that Dad might die shortly because the vein could burst and cause a fatal aneurysm. This daunting prospect led Uncle Charlie to plan one last family hurrah. It likely also explains Dad's willingness to play our silly games with such recklessness, and Uncle Charlie's tolerance of the attention that such games brought to our group.

On Aunt Jill's advice, Dad sought a second opinion in Los Angeles and the diagnosis was correct, but the outlook painted was less grim. He was advised that the vein might burst tomorrow, in six months, five years, 20 years or that he might die of natural causes that were non-AVM related. Dad was told he could keep up his daily visits to the gym and weekly tennis games but was warned never to ignore an intensely severe headache. If he experienced searing head pain, a trip to the hospital should be speedy. Mum and Dad had little choice but to hope for the best and go on with their lives. I don't know how my parents got through that summer, but they did.

—◠◡◠—

I entered Grade 8 that year with little fanfare. Apart from Phys Ed, I enjoyed school and achieved reasonable grades. Co-ed swimming classes left me terrified and like many of the girls, I did everything I could to avoid them. Trying to hide my body behind a towel, I got changed as fast as I could, while trying not to appear too dodgy. Most girls were worried about hiding their boobs in swim class and would cross their arms over their chests, hugging themselves. If they let their teeth chatter a bit they could fake being cold. What was I faking? With one hand over my chest and the other shielding my stomach, I looked like I was in some sort of pain. My anxiety would mount as I started to think about practising our dives. How was I going to execute a normal dive and then surreptitiously and speedily readjust my bag so it didn't stay flipped up and look like a balloon on my body? It was like some sort of warped agility test. I'd pop up after I'd glided under water for a few feet, then, hold my breath, go back under while I bent, rolled and flipped. Hide, hide, hide. I could exhale as soon as I knew my bag was flat again and get back in line for the next dive. I remember thinking, When can we get back to doing lengths in the pool? Physical exertion was much easier than feeling spent emotionally.

One morning, as I approached the pool's edge, I executed a crisp, smooth dive into the pool. I really stretched out. The whoosh of water running over me momentarily made me feel graceful, maybe even powerful. An image of a dolphin flashed in my brain. Ever since seeing a video with Olivia Newton-John swimming with them, I had a burning desire to do the same. Years later, I fulfilled this dream and it was as magical and exhilarating as I had hoped. But this was before then, and I wasn't a dolphin, or swimming with them. I was in a pool with horny teenage boys.

I needed to get out of the water quickly to make room for the next two divers, but I was failing my agility test and couldn't seem to get my bag in order. I had to pull myself out of the pool, floundering like a wounded seal. I looked like I was pregnant with a football. How was I going to manage this? Gus, a boy in my class, innocently commented that it looked like I had a bubble in my bathing suit. That was the final harpoon to my heart. I sped walked (no running allowed!) to the change room and sobbed in a bathroom stall. My already shaky self-esteem had just taken another hit.

Recently, while reliving my junior high school diving experiences with my cousin Paul, he asked me why I couldn't just opt out of that part of the gym class. A good question; it got me thinking back to that time. I didn't think I had the right to make the request to skip the diving. I was a girl whose body had been invaded time after time with no way to say no. I needed the tests, I needed to be cut open, I needed the needles, I needed to be in a hospital surrounded by sick children, or I would have died. I had no control over what was being done to my body and had no power to end all these horrific things. This was true not only for the deeply invasive surgeries, but also for a wide spectrum of medical exams and treatments. Sometimes I felt like a commodity that was being measured, weighed and discussed in medical jargon. Very private areas of my body were invaded regularly with fingers, scopes, tubes etc... and I had to comply. Doctors and nurses examined the physical me, but there was no professional measuring what was happening to me emotionally.

I lost my voice along the way. I thought maybe if I were quiet everything would be easier. I was like a deer in the headlights a lot of the time, frozen. Frozen, in shock and fear. I felt I was in danger, but had no place to run. It was later, through therapy, that I discussed the sensation of feeling stuck. When I was sick, there was no space in my brain to process emotional distress; I needed all of my strength to stay alive. I soldiered through the physical pain, and, as a family, we made the best of situations as they arose. I didn't investigate the lasting consequences of all these traumas until many years later.

As a youngster, I was aware that my surgeries affected others and not just me. That was a terrible burden, so I didn't voice concerns that I deemed "little things." I had a lot of perspective to draw from; worrying about swim class rated way lower on the suffering scale than being deathly ill. Also, all the other girls wanted out of swim class too, so maybe I just wanted to be like them. I don't remember my exact thoughts but I do have memories of fear. I was afraid of standing out, so not making a fuss was very important to me. I was also worried that if my peers knew the real me, they might not like me. I felt that I was too different from them, yet, on the outside I fit in.

I was a late bloomer due to the surgeries interrupting my development. When my period finally arrived, Mum and I called Aunt Jill to celebrate. She gave me the "now you're a woman" speech, which reduced the three of us to giggles on the phone. I did my best to avoid boys and was petrified of having any sort of attention drawn to me. When I was asked out on a date, I said no. One boy was so keen he asked me if I'd be ready to have a date the next year. He was trying to book six months ahead! I didn't know what to say. I had no idea if I'd be ready, but I couldn't explain why. It really was an "it's not you, it's me" situation. Poor guy. We never did go out.

In most other ways, I was an average teenager. My friend Angela and I would bike to each other's houses and talk about boys and popular music. Jane and I went to movies and would take the subway downtown to shop and hang out at the mall. My street had many kids living nearby and we would get together after dinner for large games of Kick the Can that would span over three backyards. Our ages ranged from eight to sixteen years old, so Court joined these games too. I adored my neighbourhood and the fact that we could play in the street, backyard and driveway.

Cancer

"The human spirit is stronger than anything that can happen to it."
—C. C. Scott

Aunt Jill had cancer. Mum and Dad called me into the family room and sat me down to tell me the news. I dissolved into tears immediately. Mum came over to where I was sitting alone on the contemporary, cream coloured, armless love seat and hugged me. I was just shy of fifteen and knew very little about cancer except that it killed you. How could my gorgeous, funny, creative, loving Aunt Jill have cancer? It had spread to several lymph nodes, which I knew was bad. She was going to have her right breast removed and undergo chemotherapy.

I wanted to reach out and give back some of the support she had given me. I felt helpless and too far away; I couldn't just sit and be sad, I felt driven to do something to show my aunt how much I was thinking of her. I wanted to help her, but knew there was little I could do. I called my friend Jane in tears and we walked down to The Little Party Shoppe, a store crammed with trinkets, party favours, and cards. It didn't take me long to sort through the merchandise and find what I wanted; I bought my aunt a fake dime store diamond ring and some puffy sticky letters to spell out I LOVE YOU for the card. I wrote that I wished I could send her a real diamond because I knew she liked them and that I couldn't wait to see her. Lastly, I told her to get well soon. What I didn't say was that I needed her to get better. Some people seem golden and Aunt Jill was one of these people. She loved life; if hers were taken too soon it would mean that spirit alone is not enough.

My aunt having cancer terrified me on many levels. I permitted myself to feel a personal loss that I hadn't been able to feel for myself when I was sick. It was more acceptable to me to mourn the loss of her health than my own. The dread of losing her was real and tangible. The anxiety for myself was buried underneath the "Ireland spirit" that I was told I possessed, like my grandfather. Suddenly, life seemed very unfair and scary. No one was safe. No one was protected. Not even the golden. I wanted to help her and was all too aware of her pain. Our mutilated bodies shared a badge of courage. A lopped off breast or ileostomy didn't make us less lively. We knew that the wounds themselves were superficial; we had to persevere against the diseases. The loss of one breast or an unsmooth stomach is surmountable. I just wasn't sure I could take the loss of Aunt Jill. Dad went to Los Angeles to visit and lift her spirits while she began chemotherapy.

Aunt Jill was diagnosed in the early spring of 1984, so the planned summer trip to Vermont was altered. She had always wanted to live at the beach and took her diagnosis as a way to achieve her dream. She and Uncle Charlie rented a house on Malibu Beach and invited me for my usual August visit. Like my aunt, I believe the ocean has a therapeutic healing quality and, even as her hair fell out, she shone during those months at the beach. She was tanned and fit-looking while she fought a deadly disease.

Aunt Jill read about, and practiced, alternative medicines, including the healing properties of crystals and meditation. With Katrina at ballet camp in another state, Aunt Jill led Su and me in meditation sessions. She hand picked us each crystals to hold, as well as necklaces. I loved the feel of the smooth, cool rose quartz in my palm as I closed my eyes and listened to the sound of the ocean with my aunt and cousin. We would focus on our breathing, slowly letting air in and out of our noses, and the effect was almost tribal. I felt connected to them, myself and the sea. Before I went home that summer, Aunt Jill recorded a meditation tape for me so her voice could be with me, even when she wasn't.

While living at the beach, my aunt also spent time alone on her bedroom balcony, overlooking the waves of the Pacific, imagining her healthy cells devouring her cancerous cells. When Aunt Jill wasn't absorbing the power of nature, I often saw her surrounded by lined yellow notepads and Ziplock bags full of colourful pens as she began writing to help channel her thoughts and feelings. Later, her pages and pages of thoughts became a book.

Aunt Jill wrote two books, the first when she was battling cancer, *Life Wish* and then, a few years later, *Life Lines*, which was less about her cancer and more about my grandpa's health challenges, and about my cousin Jason's battle with drug addiction. While she was writing the second book, Aunt Jill called me and asked if she could write about my operations. I said no. I didn't take time to think about it, but I was very definite in my response and she respected my point-blank answer. Her question made sense; there was a very obvious continuity in the story line between Grandpa's colostomy and my ostomy. Also, I knew sharing my experiences might be helpful to others, but I wasn't ready to take the chance that it might be harmful to me. It's only with a lot of life experience under my belt that I think the reward might outweigh the risk.

As she wrote, her creativity helped harness her fortitude as well as gratitude for the life she was living. She was a warrior and went into battle against cancer with all guns loaded. I believed in her strength and thought that if anyone was going to win, she would.

As kids we would often skinny dip in the pond in Vermont. This was always Aunt Jill's idea. We laid our big terry towels on the prickly grass and our toned, bronzed bodies soaked up the sun as we dried off from our swims. There was the lurking danger of the boys crashing our little nudist colony on their dirt bikes, but if they did, we screeched like wild monkeys in the forest and wrapped ourselves up.

This aspect of farm life lost its appeal for me after my operation. I felt a tinge of envy when I was around my cousins in their bikinis, let alone their birthday suits. It was after Aunt Jill lost her breast that I joined the nudist party again. All of a sudden there were two of us with our war wounds on display. She had refused reconstructive surgery so there was a big bold scar across her chest where her breast used to be. She was a lopsided wonder and didn't feel any less of a woman for it. I learned a lot from this and definitely felt less alone with my beat-up belly.

I wondered if she remembered her advice to hide my bag with sexy lingerie. Of course, the shopping trip was before Aunt Jill had a mastectomy, and before she publicly shared that "sex was a mind game, and Charlie still finds me sexy with one breast." She might not have thought of it that way anymore. If she'd have reflected on it, she might have said confidence is sexy, or, if a guy doesn't like your bag, it's his loss and a big loss at that.

We never spoke about it, but she continued to dress me up in her clothes and give me things that she thought looked good on me. Image was so important in her business and I think I picked up on this idea by osmosis, as well as by the Bronsons' behaviours. Aunt Jill and Uncle Charlie relied on their looks for their job, and subsequently were concerned with keeping fit, looking attractive and youthful. Aunt Jill had all the young girls join her on a diet one summer, even although none of us were the least bit overweight. The hunger seemed to be a way of connecting us, but maybe she just didn't want to be alone with that gnawing feeling. I hadn't logged any real miles as a woman yet, and wouldn't feel genuinely comfortable in my own skin for many more years.

My aunt fought her cancer like a strategic warrior. Her mental battle against the disease earned her five cancer-free years after her initial rounds of chemotherapy and radiation treatments. She desperately wanted to survive. When her cancer made an aggressive reappearance, it was as clear as her meditation crystals that she still wasn't ready to leave this earth.

Chapter 12

Good-bye

—ɯɯ—

"How lucky am I to have something that makes saying goodbye so hard."
—A. A. Milne

Saying goodbye to Aunt Jill broke my heart. I literally understood the meaning of that phrase when I saw her for the last time. My chest ached when I saw how withered she had become. Su was living in New York, so when I made the trip to see Aunt Jill in California. I stayed at the house with just her and Uncle Charlie. Paul and Val visited several times to see me over my five-day stay. By this time, my aunt and uncle had purchased and renovated a spectacular, sprawling, ranch-style bungalow situated in an exclusive gated Malibu community. Their neighbours were Mel Gibson, James Cameron and Rick Springfield, to name a few. When Olivia Newton-John said something to me in passing at the local pet store, I was so star-struck that I couldn't speak.

The second day of my visit, Aunt Jill took me into her dressing room and told me she had something to show me. She opened one of her jewelry boxes and there, amongst her gold, silver and precious gems was the $1.99 "diamond" ring that I had sent her when she was first diagnosed with cancer. She told me she kept it in the box she has on her dresser, not in the safe, because she liked the daily reminder of me. I was surprised and deeply moved by this revelation. I knew if I tried to talk I would bawl, so I carefully embraced her bony body and choked back my tears.

On the morning when I was going home, Uncle Charlie took me to their bedroom to say goodbye to Aunt Jill. I knew it would be the last time. The sun was streaming in their big bedroom windows overlooking the garden of trees and bright pink bougainvillea. The French patio doors were partially open to let in fresh air and the sounds of birds.

Aunt Jill looked small tucked in bed. Her little face was shrivelled like a newborn chick, and her head was covered in downy, fluffy, white hair. Although her soft cotton sheets and eiderdown duvet engulfed her, extra layers of soft blankets were piled on top of the bedding. A pale pink cashmere shawl was draped around her shoulders, and her gold and diamond watch looked heavy on her slight wrist. Her large diamond eternity band slid around on her finger. My aunt was soft and sparkly even as she was fading away. Were the jewels her armour? They couldn't save her. She was emaciated and still didn't accept the fact that she was dying. Her eyes were sunken and shadowed and her bones were jagged and almost exposed through her pale papery skin. I felt an overwhelming despair knowing that I would soon be leaving her, and her me, forever. I perched on the bed and she asked me why I didn't sit on the more comfortable bedside chair. Uncle Charlie quietly explained, "She wants to be close to you, Jill."

With that, she took my hand in hers, but she was not interested in a final goodbye. She was sleepy, so we didn't talk much, although, she did manage to say, "Look after Sulika; she really respects you." That was the only way I knew that she had some cognizance that this was the end.

Thirty minutes later, I was still sitting on Aunt Jill's bed when she asked me for another pillow—she gingerly propped herself up while rasping, "I want to give you some things before you leave." My aunt always gave me clothes when we were together; a few days before we had packed up two trunks of her hand-me-downs. She had given me a gorgeous black taffeta, mermaid-style ball dress, as well as a trunk full of other designer dress clothes. I had no use for these garments, but we had enjoyed the ritual of me trying them on and packing them up. This visit, Uncle Charlie sat with Aunt Jill as I gave them a fashion show of his wife's clothes. I felt like my aunt's very own paper doll, and she seemed like she genuinely enjoyed the game of being fashion director and dressing me up. I know I did. It was a slice of fun for both of us during a dark time.

My bags were already at the front door. I was horrified that Aunt Jill was trying to get out of bed to give me more. As I protested, I looked at Uncle Charlie for some guidance and he just smiled sadly and said, "Jill, is that a good idea?"

She staggered to her feet, gripped my arm and growled, "I'm fine, Charlie."

I barely remember the next few moments; I was so terror-stricken that she would die, in her vast closet, while giving me her things. She grabbed a pile of clothes that became a barrier between us as I said my final goodbye in her boudoir. During that trip she had told me she wished she could give me her car. Maybe more clothes made her feel like she was compensating for something she couldn't give me. I'm not sure. My guess is that she wanted to extend our time together. I know she wanted to extend her time on earth. She had sabotaged my departure days on previous visits. Delayed breakfast so I might miss my plane. Given me things to fit in my already full suitcase at the last minute so I was running late. Tried to convince me to stay just a day or two longer. I hated goodbyes as much, if not more, than she did—this was another thing we had in common. This time there was a lot more at stake; it was our final goodbye. We both knew it, but didn't say it. I cried the entire way to the airport and felt bereft on the flight home.

Aunt Jill was never ready to go. When her doctors continually told her it was hopeless and her body was failing her, she still ravaged her body with risky treatments, burning her throat and vocal cords in the process. She waged a brutal war, but, to the great dismay of all who loved her, six months after learning of her cancer's return, she lost the battle. I was devastated.

Chapter 13

Dr. Gaze

—⚹—

"A cat has absolute emotional honesty: human beings for one reason or another, may hide their emotions, but a cat does not." —Ernest Hemingway

Two years after graduating university with a Bachelor of Science in Psychology, I was working at a rewarding job in psychology research at The Hospital for Sick Children. It was weird to employed by the hospital where I'd first been sick all those years ago, and it was made worse when I started experiencing bouts of extreme sadness. It was during this time that my parents separated and a few years after my aunt Jill died of breast cancer, so I decided I needed some help.

I was good at compartmentalizing my sadness; productive and cheerful in the daytime, but teary after work in the evening. I would cry in the bathtub. I would cry in the car. I would cry when I was alone and feeling safe and surrounded. I was generally a positive and optimistic person, and that is how most people knew me. My distress was not apparent to anyone around me. My inner suffering was just that, inner. It was so hidden that my family doctor, who knew me well, dismissed my request for a therapist saying, "You don't need a shrink, you're the most adjusted person I know." I burst into gut-wrenching sobs and procured the name of a psychiatrist. It's supposed to be a compliment to seem well adjusted, but I knew that asking for help was the best thing I could do to assist myself in actually feeling the way people perceived me. In January 1993, I began seeing Dr. Gaze.

My parents' separation was the final catalyst to help me realize that I would benefit from a therapist. Mum and Dad had been married for about 25 years and although a great match in many ways, their partnership was no longer working as husband and wife. Courtenay had graduated high school and was travelling in New Zealand and Australia with a friend when Mum and Dad split up. Court and I were supposedly "adults," but I still felt the acute loss of our family unit. Our foursome was my foundation, and although it wasn't surprising news, the separation felt like a major blow to my stability. We had been a strong team. We were still a strong team, but fractured. I had been needy of my family so many times. How was this new dynamic going to work? I worried about Dad. He was already often left out of our estrogen party, Mars to our Venus. Now he'd be physically separated from us too.

After the decision to split had been made, things progressed quickly. When Courtenay returned home from her travels, we had a garage sale where we profited from all our Barbie stuff and kid games. Our family home was sold, and Mum, Courtenay and I moved to a new, smaller, but very hip downtown semi-detached row house. Dad first rented a condo by the lake, and then bought one closer to our old neighbourhood.

After some initial tension, Mum and Dad civilly divided their possessions and assets, somehow managing to remain amicable. It was one of the nicest breakups I have ever heard of. It was a "conscious uncoupling" before Gwyneth Paltrow made the term a new-age lifestyle phenomenon. Basically, the idea is that both people in the couple come to understand that one person is not at fault for the break-up. It's about understanding what patterns one brought to the partnership, and taking some responsibility for the breakdown of the relationship. That's the very short version of the method, as I understand it.

I am incredibly grateful that my parents' split was not acrimonious; it made it easier on Court and me. Our family still celebrates holidays and family milestones together, and comes together during a crisis. My parents have been known to play bridge together and go to the movies now and then. Mum and Dad remain friendly to this day and I don't anticipate that ever changing.

During that time in therapy, I focused a lot on how our rescue Siamese cat, Psyche, was managing with all the change in the house. I was projecting my feelings onto the family cat. In one of our sessions, I said, "Psyche is feeling lost, yowling and wandering aimlessly, because I imagine she doesn't like all the changes."

Dr. Gaze quietly asked "What else do you think she is feeling?"

"Alone and scared," I answered. "She is very clingy. She knows we are going somewhere, but isn't sure where. She's afraid we are leaving her behind."

Dr. Gaze was taking copious notes during those sessions. It wasn't hard to figure out why.

Chapter 14

Falling

—ᘱᘱ—

"We only control what we don't trust."   —Glennon Doyle

In 1993, shortly after seeking out Dr. Gaze, I began dating my future husband, Steve. We met through mutual friends. Steve worked with my good friend's brother so he was on the scene a fair bit. He liked to party and knew how to have a good time.

The girls in our group of friends loved to go dancing and the guys joined us to watch and drink beer in crowded, hot, loud, smoky bars. Steve often joked, saying, "You girls are like salmon, swimming upstream to spawn." I thought that was funny.

We were a demure group in how we dressed—jeans, flat shoes or boots, and sweaters, but we shook and shimmied to seventies, eighties and nineties songs from various genres. It was mostly a weekend ritual although, when I wasn't feeling blue, I still saw my girlfriends, after work, on weekdays for dinner, a movie, trivia night or a workout. But we were weekend warriors. It was a fun time; there was lots of laughing, flirting and camaraderie over drinks. Sometimes a bunch of us would crash at my friend's house instead of going home in the wee hours of the morning. Steve thought it was hilarious that my parents would pick me up on the Sunday morning to take me out for a family brunch. He was the youngest of four kids and this type of curbside service struck him as very high brow and odd. It was a lot better than doing the Walk of Shame to the bus, or waiting for someone with a car to wake up, so I never thought to question the arrangement.

There was an obvious attraction between Steve and me, but he was known as a bit of a "bad boy," so I was wary. The fact that he rode a motorcycle was not appealing; I couldn't see myself perched on the back of his hog, but soon after I met him, he sold that and bought a red sports car. That was only marginally more attractive—I've never liked noisy cars that are low to the ground. Other boys in the group expressed interest in me too, but they didn't hold my attention the way Steve did. Our physical attraction was intense.

Steve loved baseball and attended the home opening games of the Toronto Blue Jays each year. I was out with my girlfriends and Su (she was visiting her dad on a movie set in Toronto) when Steve and his friends met up with us at a bar, after the Jays' home opener. We all drank and cavorted the night away as the men celebrated the start of baseball season. I enjoyed dancing with my cousin and friends. Steve knew the way to this girl's heart was on the dance floor, so he courted me with his moves. I was intrigued by his somewhat aloof persona and liked that he seemed to have his own slightly alternative style. I kissed him that night, and he asked me on a date. I said yes and was excited to see him again.

He stood me up on our first date. I had taken special care with my make-up, was dressed in a tight black mini skirt and pretty cream coloured sweater, waiting for him to take me to dinner. He never showed up. My mother couldn't believe it and advised me to be done with him. He called me a couple of days later to apologize, he had been golfing, his foursome had gotten drunk, and he just forgot about me. He asked to make it up to me, but I was still stinging, so I said we would be better going out in a group.

It was an emotionally charged time for me. Like Psyche, my cat, I was needy. I had put myself on a fat-free diet and chopped off my hair for a new pixie cut. A couple of adults told me I looked like Audrey Hepburn, and I was thrilled. I wasn't consciously trying to look sick, but my body was very lean, and bordering on bony. My boyfriend before Steve asked me to gain some weight because my bones might puncture him. I was slowly disappearing. Did I want to become invisible? Or more visible, by disappearing? Illness had always garnered me lots of attention, so maybe I was ensuring that I wasn't forgotten while our family unit was being severed. Mum and Dad nagged me to gain weight, but I continued with an intense exercise regime, and claimed I no longer had a taste for butter, cheese and fatty foods.

I still have trouble loving my body. It has let me down so many times. From a very early age I couldn't trust it to be healthy. Forget about love, it's hard to like something that you don't trust. As a young adult I privately figured I would get cancer later in life, like my aunt. I expected my body to fail me again, sometime. Since my teenage years, I worked hard at being physically fit, but my goal was never "big and strong." I was always more comfortable looking thin and small.

It wasn't just my size; I kept my voice small too. Ever since I was a child, every school report card said that I needed to "speak up more in class." I would rather have stuck needles in my eyes than draw attention to myself in the classroom. Presentations just about killed me. I didn't dream big either. I had a secret desire to try acting lessons, but never waded into those waters; I told myself there was no point because I could never be an actress. What a shame, I might have enjoyed trying and learned to come out of my shell in that environment.

When I look back at my twenties and "fat-free" days, it seems clear that I was struggling and wanted a replacement for the family that I felt was disintegrating. I had lost my aunt, and saw less of my cousins and uncle. I was only seeing Dad once a week for dinner, and at the time we weren't particularly close. He had just started seeing a therapist himself, so we seemed to both be dancing around one another, trying to connect.

My sessions with Dr. Gaze were very helpful, but they were hard work and often left me feeling emotionally spent. It was difficult to relive so many horrific events from my childhood and acknowledge the fear, pain and sadness that were still within me. I was recognizing that during the times of my childhood surgeries, I often felt unseen, invisible. Doctors and nurses could see the physical me, but my emotional needs went unrecognized.

Maybe this was one of the reasons I was so attracted to Steve. Therapists will tell you that you are drawn to what you know. Steve seemed focused on my physical attributes, I could tell he liked what he saw when he looked at me, but he was more evasive emotionally. Although he had forgotten about me for our first date, Steve was persistent for a second chance; he did everything he could to make me feel special, and to let me know he wanted to see more of me. I liked his attention and was still attracted to him when we were out together partying, so we began seeing each other as a couple.

Steve was very demonstrative and loving, and that was enough for me to forgive him his weaknesses and begin falling in love with him. Steve definitely had issues with alcohol, but I was overindulging on the weekends too, so I just focused on the fact that he clearly thought I was awesome. That part felt good, it felt really good, and I needed that. He made me feel pretty the way my aunt had, and he didn't bat an eye about my ileostomy. He just thought I was sexy, period. I still kept the lace teddies in my lingerie drawer, folded, and surrounded by special scented bars of soap. They remained a symbol of my femininity, but were an unnecessary aid to my sex life.

Chapter 15

History

—〰—

"Empathy grows as we learn."   —Alice Miller

I had so much to unravel at each weekly appointment with Dr. Gaze. To make up my work hours, I stayed late twice a week so I could see her more often. Once we opened my Pandora's Box of emotions, I felt empowered by sorting through them, and learning more about how I was put together. I was figuring out where to fit the pieces of my puzzle and how it all connected. I learned that parents and their upbringing influence all of us. By talking about my mum and dad and their histories, I gained a greater insight into them, as people, as well as an appreciation of how their backgrounds affected my relationship with them and others.

My parents were raised to keep a stiff upper lip. Although not a perfect way to get through life, it did have some advantages. Instead of exploring whether things were fair, or how they would cope, they just soldiered on. They viewed things in a pragmatic way and got stuff done. I inherited that way of thinking about my surgeries. It was with Dr. Gaze that I was able to put aside some of that stoicism and take the time to examine the emotional toll of my physical traumas. I continued to be practically-minded, but I also allowed myself to take care of all my business, mind and body.

Growing up, I had a generous helping of my father's traits—I was a planner and industrious. But despite my similarities with my dad, I felt closer to my mum when I was younger. This was due in part because Dad believed in strict rules for Court and me, so we didn't get the benefit of his humorous side very often. He was very protective of us, and would try and scare us into staying on the right path. His love of acting sometimes translated into a flair for the dramatic. This, combined with fear for his girls' safety, could make for some fantastical stories.

For instance, anytime we drove by the large, impressive looking Hare Krishna church on our way downtown, he would warn us in a stern, grim voice that kids who went into that church *never came out*. Most weeks, the church had a sign posted offering a free lunch. According to Dad, the lunch actually had a very high cost. People, although he emphasized kids, who made the grave error of accepting the food were kidnapped into a cult and never saw their parents again.

He seemed deadly serious, and it was a terrifying prospect. As a family we had never been to church, so Court and I had no real reference point as to what went on inside houses of worship. My sister and I were never short of food, so it's interesting that he worried about us being tempted by their free lunches. Poor Court. Years later, one evening, when she, Su and I were playing around a small, white, steepled church in Vermont, my cousin and I jokingly told her stories of lurking spirits, and my sister peed her pants in fear. She related churches to kidnappings. As for me, until I was about twenty-five, I couldn't drive by the Hare Krishna's church without a feeling of dread.

It was after my first stay in hospital that I understood how much Dad cared about me. His rules didn't change, and he wasn't any more demonstrative with his affection, but because he had been so present for me when I was sick, I knew he loved me very much. He showed me in ways that were intuitive to him. He told me stories and talked with me during the scary nights. He always straightened up my hospital bed, and made sure my sheets were wrapped tightly around me. He neatened my flowers and cards. These things matter immensely in his tidy world, so he was doing what he understood to ease anxiety.

With Dr. Gaze, I explored how Dad's history with his own childhood made it hard for him to be outwardly affectionate with his wife and daughters. My father told me things that could have been emotionally devastating to him in a very matter of fact way. He never complained about his family, but I knew them all well and could fill in many of the blanks. He had grown up with an emotionally distant and overly competitive mother who seemingly placed more value on her daughter than her son. He had been banished to Canada. Kicked off the island. If he was insecure and unable to express his love easily, I began to understand why. He hadn't felt cherished himself. It went beyond that; he felt disposable. He had been tossed to the curb by his own family. I found empathy for him as well as compassion for his defensive behaviours.

After my parents separated, it was especially important to me to foster a relationship with my father. I began meeting him every week for dinner. At first, I did it because I felt badly for him. Mum, Court and I are were still living together and I imagined Dad was very lonely.

The more I worked with Dr. Gaze, I discovered I wasn't just meeting Dad to help him; I also yearned for a deeper relationship with him. There were lots of things that I liked about my father. If he had rejected my attempt at closeness, I would have been very hurt, but I had the benefit of all those late-night hospital chats to remind me of the depth of his love, so I decided to try and find a way to develop a shared appreciation of each other.

It wasn't always an easy process. I would bristle, and he could drive me batty when he would try and tell me what to do, or exaggerate the danger of one thing or another. Gradually, instead of taking it personally, or thinking that he thought me stupid, I understood he often forgot that I was a young adult, making a living and my own choices, and would fall back into his role as The Boss. He was comfortable in that role. He had built a successful company by being in charge, and his parents had raised the children to be seen and not heard at home. He had been taught that it was adults that commanded respect, not children.

I learned to calmly laugh about some of his ludicrous warnings, and pay attention to the ones with merit. I found ways to express myself without pushing him away. When Steve and I were planning a trip to Costa Rica, I excitedly told Dad our plans. His knee-jerk reaction was to warn me, in a raised, angry voice, "Don't go into the rain forests barefoot, the snakes can bite, and you would be too far from a hospital for an antidote. They're deadly!"

Not the reaction I had been hoping for. That would have made me exceedingly frustrated in the past, but now I knew that he was expressing his own old-fashioned protective form of love. Did he worry more about me dying because of my illnesses? Maybe. Regardless, I burst out laughing and countered with, "I think you've raised me better than to troop through the rainforest barefoot, Dad. I'm not a total idiot."

He relaxed, laughed, and then we moved on.

The more I got to know Dad, the more I appreciated his street smarts and insights. Way before the date rape drug "roofies" was common knowledge, Dad warned me to never drink anything that I hadn't seen being made. When my friend Angela and I, fake ID in hand, were hitting the adult dance clubs in our teen years, he stayed up in the living room chair making sure I got home on time. We frequented those clubs until we went to university and he was always there waiting. Dad would ground me if I was late, but really, he just wanted me home safe from all the bad guys out there that he imagined might hurt me.

I am immensely happy that I found my way to a caring, demonstrative relationship with Dad. It was worth taking the risk of being hurt. Sharing my trials and tribulations with him almost always proves beneficial, as he is a non-judgmental and smart sounding board who has an excellent grasp on human behaviour. He now expresses his love verbally to me, and we miss each other now that I am no longer living in Toronto. His old self couldn't have told me that—now he says it with ease.

Conversely, instead of finding closeness with my mother through therapy, I needed to loosen some of the stitches that had sewn us together. Among other things, Court, Mum and I share an interest in clothes, shoes, interior decorating, movies, and pop culture. Our female bond was established easily. Mum enjoyed being a mother and was involved in our young lives, driving us to our various lessons, and taking us shopping for clothes and school supplies when we needed them.

When I left for university, I knew having her eldest chickadee leave the nest was difficult for Mum, but I didn't realize until later, when Court told me, that she continued to spend a lot of time sleeping in the family room chair. She had started that behaviour when I was in high school, and it continued for several years until she separated from Dad.

She was depressed. I don't think she ever quite realized how much her mother's behaviour had affected her until she went to therapy. Even while she was talking to a therapist weekly, she didn't want to acknowledge that her mother likely suffered from mental illness. Maybe it made her too worried about her own mental health. She also avoided talking about my time in hospital with her therapist; it was too much for her to revisit that pain. It was an unhealed wound: poke at it too much and the mess would be exhausting to clean up. Watching Mum suffer through her inertia and sadness helped me understand that, when I started to feel melancholy in my twenties, I needed to seek some professional help. I instinctively knew that my sorrow wasn't a chemical imbalance; I just had some work to do.

When Mum and Dad split, Mum had withdrawn from her friends and used me as her sounding board and confidante. Mum had been seeing a therapist for several years before she and Dad separated and she and I openly talked about her childhood, and, less appropriately, her relationship with Dad. She acknowledged that her psychiatrist had told her not to share her revelations about Dad with me, but somehow, we usually ended back there. Even though I knew it wasn't healthy for me, or my relationship with my father, part of me felt honoured that Mum trusted me, and my opinion. It made me feel special. I also learned a lot about the process of therapy by listening to her. My friends marvelled at my close relationship with my mother, and I spoke to her every day while I was at university. I had been so dependent on her when I was sick that the umbilical cord was hard to cut for both of us.

I was majoring in psychology at school, so had a general interest in the science of behaviour and mind, and the study of conscious and unconscious feelings and thoughts. I didn't require a degree to understand that I needed to curtail the habit of being Mum's second therapist and pseudo marriage counsellor. Once I started seeing Dr. Gaze, I worked on developing opinions about my dad that were just that, my opinion, based on my interactions with him. I also explored Mum's emotional neediness.

She couldn't count on her mother's love and approval, and her dad had been too weak to step in when he should have, so Mum had often walked on eggshells around her mother. Once, when Mum broke up with a boy that my grandmother had hoped was marriage material, she gave my mum the silent treatment for five months. Mum lived at home at the time, and had to endure that behaviour without anyone coming to her aid, and without having other accommodation options. By this time, Uncle Gordon was becoming overly attached to alcohol, and living on his own. Unfortunately, he continued down this path until his body was so deficient in thiamine that he developed Sarkoff's Syndrome in his late twenties. This resulted in the loss of his short-term memory; his long-term memories before he became an alcoholic remained intact. It was a sad situation: no wonder Mum wanted to move far away.

As I had with my dad, through therapy, I found a new degree of empathy for Mum and understood that her relationship with Courtenay and I helped her heal from what she had experienced with her own family. She wanted to feel needed, be needed and have closeness with us that had eluded her with her mother. I have never questioned the fact that Mum enjoys my company and wants me around. Courtenay and I are her two favourite companions.

Chapter 16

Squirrelly

—◆—

"The past gets carried with us. It's always there." —Ann Pearlman

I had vivid nightmares when I first began therapy with Dr. Gaze. As well as examining my relationship with my parents, she and I discussed my childhood hospital experiences in great detail, and many suppressed feelings began to surface. Unearthing the past pain seemed to free up my psyche for horrendous dreams. I would wake in the night screaming, bathed in sweat, exhausted and terrified. After bolting upright in bed, and blinking through the darkness to establish where I was, I would find relief in the present and wait awhile before I went back to sleep, so the dream didn't reboot from where I had exited.

It is rare now that I remember my dreams when I wake up, but back then my nightmares often involved an animal that I didn't like: squirrels. My fear of squirrels began before I was sick. When I was about ten, one had tried to break through our backyard screen door and I panicked, thinking it was going to bite me. It wasn't the least bit scared of me, and didn't look like a normal skittish rodent. From the little I knew about rabies, I thought this squirrel might be infected. I got the glass door closed before he gnawed through the screen, and, once deterred, the squirrel fled. Years later, when I was at university, I awoke one night to see a black squirrel sleeping at the end of my bed, on the warm lump made by my feet. What happened next was like a scene in a cartoon. I bolted upright, shrieked, and the squirrel made eye contact with me, looked like it had received an electric shock, and zipped out the screenless window the same way I assume it came in. I placed glass bottles along my window sill from that day forward to ward off all vermin and I crossed the street if I came upon one near the sidewalk. My fear of squirrels was featured prominently in one particularly vile nightmare.

Everything was dark, I couldn't see very well, like a horror movie. My hair was ratty and unkempt; I looked dirty, uncared for, and homeless. I was walking through an overgrown forest, navigating through tall grasses and prickly scrub. I knew there were no other humans in the untamed wildlife all around. I was on high alert for predators and wished I had night vision goggles. I grew jumpier and more anxious every time I looked over my shoulder.

I felt exposed, with no weapons and very little clothing. I was covered in goosebumps, wearing only thin, loose cotton gray pajama pants and a threadbare, short-sleeved t-shirt. I had on sandals that were just soles of leather with one tenuous strap attaching them to my feet. I shuffled rather than walked, clinging to the bottoms of my shoes with my clenched toes so they didn't fall off. I took a big step up to begin walking on a crumbled stone wall so I could have a better view of what was ahead. It was like a very wide balance beam, and I had to concentrate to ensure that I didn't lose my footing. Looking around, I froze in terror.

Slowly, black squirrels with red beady eyes seemed to hatch from the ground until the surrounding earth was teeming with them. They ran around angrily and were frothing at the mouth, screeching up at me. I knew they had rabies and wanted to infect me with their small, sharp fangs. There were so many of them, how could I win? They began trying to jump up on the wall. I knew the exit to the forest was up ahead and I began to run. In desperation, I kicked off my leather soles and continued on, barefoot.

The wall was rocky and unstable, and several times I lost my footing. My feet became scraped, stinging and bloody. I didn't call for help—I knew there was no one there. With each fumble, squirrels attached to my pant leg and managed to climb onto the wall. I tried in vain to kick them off. I wasn't strong enough to fight them all. Their claws tore my skin as they pulled themselves higher.

Quickly my shaky wall was swarming with the evil, diseased squirrels. I was surrounded. They wanted to contaminate me with their rabies and eat me alive, as I slowly died an excruciating death. They began viciously gnawing at my ankles, then scraping and gnawing on my knees and calves. Blood was dripping down my body and soaked my shredded pants, and just as the black beasts got near my genitals, I woke with a blood-curdling scream.

Dr. Gaze helped me understand the emotions that were coming to the surface in my dreams. I looked homeless and felt alone in the dream. This seemed to correspond to feelings about my parents splitting up. I had just lost my family home, and more importantly, family unit. In the nightmare I was alone. Although I had the support of my family, I had been solitary in my hospital bed and in the operating room many times.

The rabies and rabid squirrels signified my bowel disease. The squirrels, like my disease, had been stronger than me and the treatment. It had always been an unfair fight, and one I didn't win until I lost my colon. There was a lot of blood, pain and fear associated with my surgeries, and there had been times I was aware that I was dying.

I awoke from the dream as my genitals were under attack; this seemed related to me being sick during my puberty years, as well as the effect on my self-esteem as a young woman. I didn't see the squirrels attack my vagina, but they wanted to. Maybe I woke up because even my subconscious wasn't ready to rip open my perceived loss of femininity. I told Dr. Gaze that I thought trying to escape the squirrels was connected to the helplessness I felt as a young child in hospital. Shaky walls, shaky ground. I knew what that felt like.

It took many months for the nightmares to stop. Despite the fact that they served as an excellent tool for dissecting my emotions, I was so happy to be rid of them.

Steve was always slightly suspicious of my therapy, or more likely, threatened by it. He thought therapists were for spoiled Hollywood types. I knew better. I continued seeing Dr. Gaze weekly. For a while, I saw her twice a week.

In my first year of therapy, I slowly started to shed many of my defensive, stoic ways. It was like taking part in an archaeological dig, unearthing and examining so many buried feelings. Many of my perceptions of the past needed dusting off for investigation. Sometimes it was an overwhelming sadness that we explored, other times, anger. Almost always, the feelings brought to the surface were intense. It didn't take me long to understand that the mantra of "my childhood surgeries made me stronger" was only a very small part of the truth. In reality, psychotherapy tapped into a strength that was much more useful than the immense energy required to haul around a heavy bundle of old pain and suffering.

I felt very proud of the work that Dr. Gaze and I did then, and still do. When people say they think I'm brave, it's not for what I consider to be my bravest moments. I had no other option than to get better when I was sick in hospital, or to do the best I could with my health challenges, but I definitely had a choice on whether or not to drag myself through all the muck of the past. Bravery to me was the fortitude and strength required to have an honest look at my life and take the road less travelled.

Chapter 17

Married!

—∿∿—

"A wedding is an event, but marriage is a life."   —Myles Munroe,
Waiting and Dating

On a trip to Cuba, around Valentine's Day in 1995, Steve proposed to me on the beach. There was no one else around; most people had disappeared to their rooms, or gone for dinner. The sun was disappearing for the day and the sky was golden. It's one of my favourite times of day on a sun-filled holiday. He didn't get down on one knee and didn't have a ring yet, but we were snuggled on a beach chair, tropical drinks in hand, when he asked if I would marry him. It wasn't out of the blue; we had discussed the future, but in no great detail. I happily said yes and Steve told me he wanted me to pick my own ring so he could be sure that I'd like it.

Like my father had been while I was growing up, Steve was emotionally distant and overly protective. I was used to that so it felt comfortable. Steve was also very affectionate, cuddly and proud of me, and that made me feel special, as my mother had. I was excited to start a new chapter of my life with Steve and ignored any warning signs that the relationship might not be strong enough to last a lifetime. I wanted to be a mother with a new family of my own. In retrospect, I wanted to replace what I felt was lost by my parents' separation.

When we got home, my mum was shocked and disappointed that I would be moving out of her house sooner than she had anticipated. I'd been out of the house while at university, but I'd always come back when I wasn't at school. Getting married meant that I'd be out of the house for good, and I don't think Mum had expected the engagement, and wasn't ready to come to terms with me moving out. Dr. Gaze, who never outwardly reacted, definitely raised an eyebrow before asking me my feelings about the news. I was happy and stuck to that. I forged ahead with wedding plans, only mildly questioning my decision once or twice, and not with Dr. Gaze. I kept those moments to myself because they didn't happen often. I was excited about the prospect of starting our own family and nesting in our own place.

I assumed that we would grow together and build a safe and secure home for ourselves, and any children that might come along. I had no doubt that Steve loved me. I felt prized. Sometimes it verged on feeling like a thing he felt proud to display, but I pushed that feeling aside.

—ɯ—

I don't remember being nervous on our wedding day. That seems a bit strange now. I was making the biggest commitment of my life, and I was in it for the long haul, and I didn't have any nerves. Our relationship wasn't perfect, but I guess I knew perfection didn't exist and I was very focused on the celebration. I was really excited. I loved having family and friends together to celebrate with us and couldn't wait for the party.

Mum had been my go-to person to help choose the venue, invitations, flowers, menu, bridesmaids' outfits and my dress. She helped with the finishing details so I didn't have to, allowing me to enjoy the lead-up time to my big day. I knew how I wanted my dress to look, but was never going to be wasteful and spend a fortune on a designer gown. After visiting a few boutiques with Mum and Court, my maid of honour, I found my dream dress at the discount store, The Bridal Factory. I bought my shoes and veil there too, so they threw in the garter. We got everything for less than $1,000. Done and done. I practically skipped out of the store.

The dress looked like raw silk, with a fitted bodice and full skirt. The top was off the shoulder with rosettes around the neckline. It was demure, pretty, accentuated my waist, and exposed my upper back, shoulders and upper chest. That was alluring enough for me. The veil clipped into the back of my hair and fell down my back to my waist. When I look at photos now, I am struck by how young I look, and I still love that dress. It was tasteful, feminine and perfect for the time.

My six bridesmaids gathered at my mum's house to have their hair and makeup done and take some pre-wedding pho-

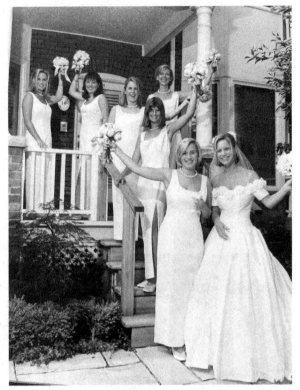

Me and my bridesmaids. *From top left:* Laura, Jen, Suzy, Angela, Su, Courtenay, and me. July, 1996.

tos. The professional makeup artist was a family friend and her work was phenomenal. It was her wedding gift to me to make us the best version of ourselves. I was thrilled with the results.

It was a hen party as we all unwrapped our dresses, admired the bouquets and tried on our shoes. Living in New York, Su hadn't been available for any fittings so we used a couple of hidden safety pins to secure her into her dress. She was in a punk rock band at the time, so it was all the more appropriate. She wasn't accustomed to looking so girly and formal, but she's naturally tall, thin and gorgeous, so, for my benefit, she wore it all with style and grace.

I wanted to be married in a garden, under the trees, and I got my wish. The day started out cloudy, but there wasn't even a drop of rain all day, and the weather improved by the hour, with perfect blue skies for our ceremony. The ceremonial garden was set up with white chairs and lush flower urns near the podium. Mum has a knack for floral arrangements and had chosen all my favourites: pale pink peonies, hydrangea and roses. Planet Earth provided the leafy trees, green grass, blue skies, bright sunshine and wispy white clouds for the rest of our set decorations.

I felt like I was starring in my own movie. A string quartet played in the corner. The bridesmaids were the first to walk down the aisle and I had chosen off-white long simple sheath dresses for them. Steve's six-year-old niece, Kristin, was the flower girl. She was a beautiful, blonde vision, wearing a pretty pink taffeta dress that Aunt Jill had given Courtenay years before. Kristin tossed pale pink rose petals down the aisle like she was made for the job. Mum wore an ivory, custom-fitted, Mother of the Bride outfit that accentuated her slim figure and had a top encrusted with a bit of sparkle and pearls. She looked fantastic. The scene was everything I had imagined.

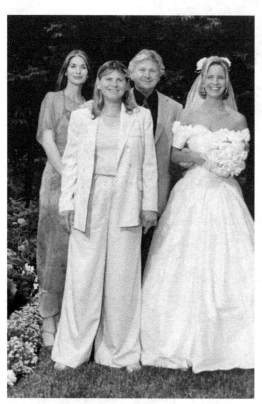

Kim, Suzanne, Uncle Charlie, and me. July, 1996.

So many of our friends and family were able to attend the wedding, including my cousin Val and his wife Shelli, my cousin Suzanne, and Uncle Charlie with his girlfriend, Kim. Uncle

Charlie cried as Dad walked me down the aisle, or maybe it was Su looking so lady-like that touched him. My guess is that he loved seeing us together, grown up, healthy and beautiful. He must have wished Jill were there for this family milestone. I know I did.

Aunt Jill had always been the one to organize family events so, when she died, I worried that Uncle Charlie would lose interest in her side of the family. But he didn't, and I trusted his love for me more than ever when in April 1993, soon after I met Steve, my Uncle Charlie contacted me because he was coming to Toronto to film a made-for-TV movie, *Family of Cops*. Su took the opportunity to visit him and spend some time with me too. She flew in for a long weekend, and we would meet up with her dad for a meal and then go do our own thing while he worked on the movie set. It was great having them in the city. He often looked wistful when we were together; I knew he had adored my aunt, and the void left by his late wife's absence would never be filled. He also probably missed our family gatherings.

Dad, Court and I had visited Uncle Charlie two months before Steve and I got married, and he gave me a pair of Aunt Jill's diamond drop earrings, which I decided to wear on my wedding day. He chose them for that reason and I was touched. He did thoughtful things like that. On my first trip back to Los Angeles after Aunt Jill died, I was with my dad, and Uncle Charlie took the two of us to her little beach house where she used to write and meditate. He hadn't changed anything in the house. It was like she had just left it to go shopping. I was swallowed up by the shabby-chic white couch, overlooking the ocean, between my dad and uncle, and quietly sobbed. I felt her there and missed her so much. No one said anything, or touched each other. We all had our time for reflection, but I suffered openly. After a while, as we were gazing outside, Uncle Charlie got up, quietly put his hand on my shoulder, and said, "I thought you'd like to come here." Then we all stood up and left.

That day, I was reminded of the first Christmas after I had my ostomy surgery, when he had taken me aside while opening our gifts and said he had something special he had chosen, just for me. He placed a small velvet box in my hands. When I opened it there was a fine gold chain with small oval gold shapes every few inches. I put the pretty chain around my neck. Uncle Charlie explained that the gold bits were actually a magnetic form of gold and were supposed to promote good health. Even Uncle Charlie, known as Mr. Tough Guy, believed in the power of hope. I wore the chain every day until about a year and half later when it got tangled in my swimsuit straps and the clasp broke. It was several years later before I had it repaired.

—ɯ—

The wedding was a fabulous party. Having so many friends and family there to celebrate with us put me on Cloud Nine. Val, Su and Uncle Charlie came up to me separately during the festivities to tell me that I reminded them of Aunt Jill. They mentioned the look of my shoulders, my back, as well as my mannerisms, smile and love of life. I wished she were there with us; she loved a good party, especially with family. Mum, Dad, Court and I had enjoyed several New Year's Eve bashes she had thrown in Vermont. I have memories of Dad dancing energetically and swirling my mum and aunt around the floor. He did the twist with me, Court and my cousins. We were a family that loved to dance together at special occasions.

Uncle Charlie left with Kim and Suzanne after the first couple of songs, Su had ditched her heels after dinner and was wearing her motorcycle boots while chatting up Steve's friend, and the rest of the guests were in full party mode. A family friend, who was my parents' former neighbour, was break-dancing in the middle of the floor. I had changed into a short, white, fitted satin dress and Steve and I danced together for the final song, Stairway to Heaven, and, as I looked across the crowded dance floor, I saw our handsome, young friend, Woody, feeling up my mother, caressing her backside. "Stairway to Heaven" is an epically long song so this was not a slip of his hand, it was a full-on, high school style grope. Mum got a good ego boost, and he got some cheap thrills. I couldn't have asked for a better celebration and the night went by way too fast.

Chapter 18

6C again

—⁓⁓—

"That's too coincidental to be coincidence."   —Yogi Berra

My therapy sessions with Dr. Gaze became even more intense when my workspace at SickKids moved from an office building outside the hospital, to within the hospital. The move was unexpected and deeply unsettling. Although I had been working for SickKids, I rarely went inside the hospital building. I was stunned to find out that our four new offices were going to be located on the 6th floor in an old ward. That ward was none other than 6C, the same one where I had been during my first hospital stay. Seventeen years later, why was the universe putting me back there? The office move impacted me profoundly. The bar was raised on the psychotherapy I had been doing with Dr. Gaze.

There were still hospital rooms just down the hall from our four Psychology Research offices. All those years later, the offices were just converted patient rooms, so the hospital loudspeakers remained in each of our offices. We could regularly hear the nurses paging one another, Code blues and all.

The walls were the same paint colours as years before. Looking at the pale mint green and yellow walls could make my stomach lurch and do weird little flip-flops. The windows and drapes hadn't changed either. Large, floor-length swaths of thick pastel-coloured fabric hung from the ceiling on narrow metal tracks, and the sound of scraping metal when they were being pulled open or closed gave me goosebumps. How many times had matching drapes been drawn around my bed so I could be examined? I'd lie there, cold and exposed, and wonder what part of me they would be investigating. I would usually look at the ceiling, or my mum, not the doctors. I knew I was a teaching instrument for the residents and I would listen to them talk about my case, and when they were done with me, minutes later, I'd hear them move on to the next child. It was a cattle call, and I was the cow, or actually, the calf. No wonder I had a complicated relationship with my body. It wasn't just the bag—I had been a human textbook, opened and closed by medical students.

The next stop on my gruesome tour of *6C Revisited* was our new coffee/lunch room. It was the former playroom where I had been wheeled for brief "outings." I had only been there a couple of times, and hadn't liked it. I felt like I was being delivered to a dilapidated clubhouse for little kids, and I didn't want to be a member. I was almost old enough to babysit the other children in the room, and in my sorry state that wasn't going to happen, so after a couple of minutes I would politely ask to go back to my room. I knew I had no energy for new friends, "playtime," or reading books, so I catalogued it as a disappointing attempt at offering me a change of scenery. It was another example of misguided good intentions, this time by a nurse.

There were so many memory vignettes that surfaced during this period of my therapy. As Dr. Gaze and I dug deeper into my trough of realizations, I began to suffer from spontaneous sweats at work. I was never exactly sure what triggered them; there were too many familiar stimuli, and memories to choose from, to be sure. I think the smells and the loudspeaker were the worst. It was like being in a time warp, a very unpleasant one.

I mainly worked at a desk on my computer, and I started having the sensation that I was very heavy, that there was lead in my shoes and I couldn't move. Not all the time, but several times a day I felt I was being sucked into my chair and had a hard time lifting myself out of it. My desk chair was well padded and on wheels so, instead of getting up, I would often roll myself over to the printer and back to my desk instead of taking the five steps required. That's how tired and stuck I felt. I felt trapped too. When I had been sick, my bed was on wheels, and I was often taken away in that, or on a gurney for medical tests or surgery. There were also times when a wheelchair had transported me around the hospital.

Dr. Gaze and I talked about how it had felt to be a young girl, deathly ill, confined to bed and immobile. It was very hard to recall what I had felt when I was a kid; I think I was on autopilot a lot of the time. As an adult processing the sensations I was experiencing, I felt waves of grief pummelling me against the shore, and would leave our sessions with red-rimmed eyes, exhausted. It was emotionally depleting doing our work, but I felt a depth of inner strength like never before.

I didn't let the hospital memories take over my headspace. I mostly enjoyed my job and colleagues. To counter feeling glued to the chair, and keep things light, I would challenge my co-worker, Min-Na, to chair races to the door or printer. I was pretty fast, but sometimes she won. We would both laugh at our absurd "racetrack". We were like kids with our snacks and would swap treats that we brought, or bring extras for each other. We both administered cognitive tests on children with diabetes and tallied their results, and sometimes we would do the tests on each other. Min-Na was clearly amazed, and perplexed, by how badly I did on the facial recognition test. It didn't occur to me that I may have a problem neurologically. I was just bad at recognizing people. It gave me a good excuse when I innocently walked by an acquaintance, or friend, on the street.

I had a weekly lunchtime appointment with Dr. Gaze during this time. We continued to dissect my inertia at the office. We explored what was causing what seemed like delayed Post-Traumatic Stress Disorder (PTSD). I was feeling stuck. Not just stuck, but worn out and slow-witted too. Drugged. The hospital halls were still noisy, and the calls over the loudspeaker were an assault to my senses and memory. Sometimes the sounds felt far away as they had when I had been dopey on anaesthetic and Demerol. My senses were overloaded from the familiar stimuli. The hospital smell reminded me of watching the cleaners in my sick rooms and them averting their eyes from me. Had I been that scary to look at or were they being polite? They mopped and wiped and moved on to the next room. It had felt like an animal at the zoo, with zookeepers picking up my waste and throwing away my scraps.

Dr. Gaze thought it had been interesting that I chose to work at The Hospital for Sick Children in the first place and now I was beginning to wonder if she was right. She would circle back to this a few months later and suggest that my wedding venue of choice was not a coincidence either. I had picked the Vaughan Estates, which was part of the Estates of Sunnybrook Hospital. She may have been taking that part too far. The Vaughan was not even visible from the hospital and the grounds and dining room were beautiful. There are not many places in the city where we could get married outside in a garden and have a lovely reception area close to home. I agreed with Dr. Gaze on most of her associations, but I'm still not sure about that one. If it was about feeling safe, being in 6C again was not my choice and did not bring back feelings of safety. As far as wedding venues, Toronto is loaded with hospitals so I don't think I subconsciously needed to be linked to one, but who knows? She was usually spot on with these things.

I had been questioning whether I wanted to continue my career in Psychology Research, and I think the move to 6C may have provided me with the motivation I needed for a change. I began taking night time courses at Ryerson University and earned a degree in fashion merchandising. I left SickKids and began working at Holt Renfrew, a high-end Canadian department store.

Chapter 19

Dump the stump

—ɯ—

"While you are experimenting, do not remain content with the surface of things." —Ivan Pavlov

Two years after Steve and I married, I began having a mucous discharge from my bum. This wasn't painful, but it was bothersome. I couldn't control it and sometimes there was a lot of leakage. It was my first issue connected with my ostomy that I had to deal with as an adult, without my parents, and I decided to go and get it checked out. The transition to making my own medical assessments and appointments was delayed because I had remained a patient at SickKids about three years longer than "normal." Did this make it any easier for me? I'm not sure, but, theoretically, I was a bit more mature.

I continued seeing my childhood surgeon until I was twenty-one. When Mum and I went for my yearly follow-up appointments, I appreciated that Dr. Filler always asked after my aunt as he had met her several times, and that he and my parents had run into each other at fundraisers, and in airports, so they still seemed connected. Dr. Filler was the Chief Surgeon at SickKids and had always made me feel seen, not like cattle, and I felt safe with him. He had a lot of patients, but at the time, I was the youngest at the hospital to ever have had the ostomy surgery, and I knew I wasn't just a case number—he remembered me. This proved to be true many times. I've run into him and his wife around the city over the years and we always have a nice catch-up chat. But by the time I reached my twenties, the time had come (and gone and then come again) when Dr. Filler had to recommend that I have follow-ups at an adult hospital.

I was referred to Mount Sinai Hospital and acquired a new surgeon and gastroenterologist. I liked them both. They weren't Dr. Filler, but I was comforted by the fact that he was close by. He had saved my life and had demonstrated his kindness often.

As an adult, I desperately wanted to avoid surgery. I tried to get the mucous under control via enemas. Every night I would shoot a prescribed solution into my rectum and then lie on my side squeezing my butt cheeks to retain the medicated liquid. I held it in for an hour trying to heal my old leaky bit of leftover bowel. I remember watching Ellen DeGeneres' stand-up routines to pass the hours. She wasn't really famous yet but I found her very funny. She made me laugh so hard that I couldn't hold the liquid in my ass, so I found other ways to pass the time.

Sometimes, I brought one of my well-loved Princess Diana books to the bedroom and looked at the photos while I passed the time. They never got old for me. Throughout my teens, Aunt Jill had continued to grow my collection, and I held on to them. Diana had died the summer before and I grieved her loss with the rest of the world. I had been glued to the TV waiting to hear if she had survived the car crash in Paris. It was unbelievable to me that she was dead. Another shining light gone. I'll never forget how quiet the city was the morning after her death. Toronto was like a ghost town as I made my way to work that day. I worked in the millinery department at Holt Renfrew and it seemed appropriate to be surrounded by fancy hats as my mind was filled with Princess Di.

I didn't give up easily; I kept at this enema routine for months, but to no avail. The annoying discharge continued to randomly leak from my bottom. The enemas did not lessen the output and they were not a fun addition to my evening. The only solution was to surgically remove my rectal stump. The stump was only there in case I wanted to try the reconnection surgery again and lose my bag. No one was telling me I had a great chance of success this time. I also knew, through my old hospital friend, Linda, that being "hooked up" posed its own set of problems. Even if the surgery was successful, which I considered unlikely, I would be back to diaper rashes, pads and leakage. Instead of mucous, the leakage would be poo.

After a bit of thought, I determined that the stump should go, and the bag could stay. Forever. No going back. Once the bit of bowel was gone, the deal was done. I was okay with that. Steve never thought I would be without a bag, so he was fine with it. I think my parents had long ago given up the thought that I would be bag-free.

I talked to Dr. Gaze about my fears of having surgery. The doctors said it would be easy, but I had never experienced a smooth surgery. I always ended up with an infection or complication. I felt that my immune system rebelled against surgery, so I was worried what this one would bring.

Whatever happened with this operation, I would be dealing with it as an adult. That was a first for me. My new surgeon didn't have the same compassionate bedside manner as Dr. Filler, but I knew she was an excellent doctor. That's what mattered the most. I liked her forthright nature. She was very matter of fact, and explained things well. She came highly recommended by Dr. Filler, which meant a lot too.

I think Aunt Jill was with me on my first appointment with my new surgeon, or at least her spirit was lurking about so that our hospital history wouldn't be forgotten. As I anxiously sat in the waiting area, the secretary called for one patient after the next. I had arrived early, but I knew it was almost my turn.

The lady behind the desk clearly called "Jill."

No one looked up. I lifted my eyes from the waiting room magazine. I had a feeling she was calling me, but I wasn't going to answer to the wrong name.

She raised her voice, again calling, "Jill!" It seemed Jill had left the building. Or, had she? "Jill Ireland!" I thought so, she meant me.

I got up and walked to the desk. "I think you are calling me, Lindsay Ireland."

She gave me a huge smile and apologized with a stream of words, "Oh my goodness, yes, there was an actress Jill Ireland, she was so pretty, but died of breast cancer and I thought of her when I saw your name . . ."

I smiled back and replied "No problem." This scenario has happened to me about three times in my adult life at doctor appointments.

My aunt wasn't that famous, so it's a bit weird, but strangely comforting.

As an adult, I went to most of my hospital appointments by myself. I would get very tense and nervous as I entered the building. Usually, I would start to perspire heavily. When I worked at SickKids, I would walk over from my job, because Mount Sinai Hospital was across the street, and when my time with the doctor was finished, I went straight to the nearby mall, found the best sale rack, and bought myself something. I reasoned that I would train myself like Pavlov's dog, and reward my scary appointments with a new article of clothing. Over time, I thought, hospital engagements would become less connected to misery and more related to something new that made me feel good. I continued this practice for several years, and eventually the massive sweats stopped. I think that it was more to do with Dr. Gaze than with my attempt at Pavlovian training. But either way, things became easier.

That winter, I booked my date for surgery, as well as some extra therapy sessions. At least this time, when I was scared, I was talking about it. It helped alleviate the stress and worry. I booked some sick time at Holt Renfrew, hoped I would be back in a few weeks, and forged ahead with my pre-op appointments.

On the day of surgery, my parents and Steve accompanied me to the hospital. Steve was allowed to come down to the surgical waiting area and he did. He looked terrified. He had never been in a hospital before, let alone the surgical area. I was scared too, but, like a recording on a loop, all I kept thinking was, I hope all the doctors and nurses involved in my procedure are well rested and have had their morning coffee. When the nurse came to wheel my bed to the operating room, Steve's eyes were misty as he said, "Take good care of her" and let go of my hand as I was taken away.

I was naked, except for a pale blue hospital gown that I had wrapped around me backwards and tried to tie up at the front. It was way too big for me, so I knew I might become uncovered. I was transferred to the cold operating table, covered with a thin sheet, hooked up to an IV and monitoring tubes, and left alone with the anaesthesiologist for a briefing. For no medical reason, he decided to pull the sheet and gown back to reveal my left breast while he told me he would be the one putting me to sleep.

I was used to being examined, but in the past, my doctors only uncovered what they needed to see. I was a sitting duck on that table; completely vulnerable. As a patient, I always wanted to be seen as a person, but this interaction left me feeling more distressed rather than feeling invisible. The saying "be careful what you wish for" comes to mind. I felt more objectified than I ever had as a child. Back then, my private areas had been exposed to a lot of doctors, most of them male, but I had never worried about them seeing me sexually. I was shocked to be facing this new and unpleasant situation, especially during an already terrifying moment. This was long before #MeToo and I did not have the wherewithal to ask him to cover me back up as my erect nipple lay exposed for his viewing pleasure. As he left the room, a nurse returned, looked disgusted and covered me up while saying, "I'm so sorry, sweetie."

She seemed kind, just like the nurses at SickKids. I knew I wouldn't be alone anymore as the preparations for surgery got underway so I put the anesthesiologist out of my mind—I had bigger concerns to consider. Lying on the operating table as an adult was different than being a child. I was anxious about human error. I wasn't as naïve. I knew surgeons weren't robots; they had fights with their spouses, or a bad night's sleep. I silently hoped my doctor was in top form that day. Then I braced myself for what lay ahead as I stared up at the big, bright, blinding operating room light. I didn't need my vision to know what came next. I knew I was in for pain, tubes, and possible complications.

—⁂—

I woke up from surgery with some intense hallucinations. I thought I was in a disco, and having a really fun night out. It felt so real. The painkiller of choice was no longer Demerol. I was connected to a morphine pump that I could control myself. Maybe being an adult patient wasn't so bad?

Beside me was an overweight, bitchy roommate who was recovering from some sort of abdominal surgery. On my second day of recovery, our doctor came in to check on us both. She visited my bed first and partially pulled the curtain around us. While I was being examined, I heard the grump in the bed beside me say, for no reason, "Ileostomies are so disgusting."

She wasn't in our sight line, and no one had addressed her, so the comment was totally unsolicited and I couldn't believe it. I didn't even know this person. My surgeon and I looked at each other and she registered the hurt on my face. Without skipping a beat, my quick-thinking doctor loudly said, "Your recovery is going so well due to the fact that you are trim and fit. It's so much harder to cut through layers of fat and it's harder for the body to heal."

I appreciated what she was doing; it felt like a victory. I smiled inwardly. She then had a terse visit with bitch face and left. I felt defended and protected. Maybe she was more like Dr. Filler than I had thought.

Once discharged, I didn't initially go home. I went to recover at Mum's house because Steve was at work from 7:30 am to 5 pm each day. He came to visit me after work and then went home, or out with the boys. I only planned to stay at Mum's for four or five days, or until I was capable of getting around a bit and making my own meals. Dad had said he would pop in on me daily once I was home, so I wasn't worried about leaving Mum's house.

As I had feared, my recovery ran into complications. My wound was exceptionally sore and not healing. I went to see my surgeon and the examination was excruciating. As I lay on my side on the narrow table, with my buttocks on display, there was no way to stifle the screams as my doctor prodded at my wound. I broke the sound barrier that day. She apologized, and I went into something like shock. The room suddenly felt fake and small, like I was in a doll's house, but I was a voodoo doll, not Barbie. My mum looked ghostly white as she helped me off the table and back into my sweat pants. We went to schedule a day surgery for the next morning. My wound was infected, and had to be reopened, drained and packed with metres of ribbon-like surgical gauze.

Thus began a six-month recovery period at home. Twice a day, home care nurses visited, changed the packing in my wound, and monitored my progress. I had repeat nurses and we developed a rapport of sorts over the months. My favourite nurse, Sue, confided that she was pregnant. I had the pleasure of watching her stomach grow over those months and feel her baby kick. Many years later, I was at a neighbourhood party and ran into Sue again. She lived around the corner from our new house. I recognized her voice at first, but couldn't place her. She had a view of my backside for the majority of my house calls, so I had listened to her, more than seen her, and she was back to her pre-pregnancy weight as her baby was now eight years old. It took me a few minutes to place her and then we laughed about her knowing me "inside and out." We realized Sue was also the nurse at my son's new school. We still keep in touch a bit.

During the weekdays Dad visited me to make sure I wasn't lonely, the laundry was done, the house was tidy, and that I had good meals to eat. He bustled about and entertained me with lively banter about his friends, and fitness club gossip. We shared some good laughs. As I slowly got better, he accompanied me on short walks around the block to help increase my strength, offering me his arm when I needed it. Around that time, my dad also drove me to my weekly appointment with Dr. Gaze and waited for 45 minutes in the car while I worked through how my situation now reminded me of other times when my health was compromised. I sat on my special donut cushion as I talked about my frustrations of still being bed ridden and weak. I could manage the boredom; it was my subconscious connections to disappearing and death that were rattling me.

As my incision healed, the length of the packing gauze decreased bit by bit. It was painstakingly slow. The difference wasn't measurable daily, but weekly. At about the halfway point, in what felt like a never-ending recovery, Dad arranged for an esthetician to come to the house and give me a manicure and pedicure. It made me feel like a young woman again, instead of a patient. It was a perfect gift!

During this time, Mum took a much-needed three-week holiday. She had booked it knowing she would need a break after my surgery. She had not planned for my infection and delays. Seeing me back in hospital had been mentally exhausting for her. It brought back many old fears from my childhood stays in hospital. Revisiting those worries was too much for her to handle. She didn't cancel her plans. Mum realized that she still needed to get away, even though my recovery had hit a bump. She knew that I had support. Now that I am a mother myself, I think I understand. Seeing your young child at the brink of death would be horrifically frightening. Even though I recovered, those memories are ones that Mum still can't talk about without welling up. At the time, I felt angry that Mum could leave me, but I was hardly alone.

Dad was an excellent caretaker. Courtenay and her then boyfriend, Brian, visited me often after work and on weekends. My friends checked in. Steve was around too. I read a lot of books over those months. I eagerly devoured some thick bestsellers that had daunted me when my life was busy.

It was a long haul, but almost six months later, I finally got back to work, and regular life. When I tried to resume my usual workouts, I found I could no longer maintain stamina on the Stairmaster. My legs quickly felt weak and shaky. I found that curious, but didn't worry about it too much. I just did the treadmill instead, as well as work with some weights.

I was glad to be back in shape and at work again, and partying on the weekends. It was a good thing I dusted off my dancing shoes because a couple of months later, Courtenay, Brian, Steve and I were invited to a party in Malibu to celebrate Uncle Charlie's marriage to his girlfriend, Kim. They put us up at the Malibu Beach Inn hotel, just 15 minutes from Uncle Charlie's home and the party venue was Wolfgang Puck's restaurant, Granita. I used my staff discount at Holt Renfrew to buy a pretty, slinky, beaded black dress and was excited to see my uncle and cousins. My sister and I booked a rental car (appropriately, a Chevy Malibu) and didn't make any plans except to see family.

The night of the party felt a bit strange. Seeing Uncle Charlie host a party without my aunt felt wrong, but I downed some champagne to numb my discomfort. I was introduced to the actors Sean Penn and Geoffrey Rush, and danced with the model, Rachel Hunter. As I was taking a break from the dance floor a woman struck up a conversation with me. The music was loud, but I swore she said she was the wife of Dr. van Schaik, Aunt Jill's riding instructor. I didn't think he'd still be alive, he was pretty old when I was a kid. She looked a bit confused as we chatted about something, perhaps Vermont, and then she said, "Oh, there he is now" and pointed directly at Dick Van Dyke, apparently a neighbour of my uncle's. Sorry, Mrs. Van Dyke, I had my aunt on the brain.

Chapter 20

Scar tissue

—∿∿—

"You may have to fight a battle more than once to win it." —Margaret
Thatcher

In the early part of 2001, I decided to see a fertility specialist. Steve
and I had been trying to have a baby, but with no luck. Mum accompanied me to my first appointment with the fertility doctor, and we
listened carefully as she laid out some of my potential options.

The doctor thought that all my surgeries had probably resulted
in a lot of scar tissue in my abdomen and around my ovaries. Having
surgery to open my belly and investigate the amount of scar tissue
was one route that I could take. During surgery, if they found tissue blocking the route to the fallopian tubes they would be unable
to take it out in the first operation. For reasons that weren't exactly
clear, they would have to let me heal and go in again to remove it. I
didn't even consider that choice. I made it clear that I wanted to avoid
drugs if possible, as well as anything remotely resembling surgery, so
our options were limited.

The first step we decided on was having my blood taken during the time when ovulation should occur, to enable the doctor to
pinpoint my most fertile day. On the day when my hormone levels
were just right, the nurse would call to advise me to *make love* within
24 hours. The entire process would take the guesswork, and romance,
out of the baby-making process. But I decided having my blood monitored would be fine. Steve didn't seem to want to be involved with
the appointments or decisions, but he did concur that he didn't want
me cut up. He agreed that my body had been through enough.

From Day 9 to the ovulation day of my cycle, I would go to the clinic by 7:30 am to have my blood taken. The dreary, windowless, waiting room was always full of women and couples. The chairs were close together, and generally the men fidgeted and looked uncomfortable, while the women were still and grim. It hadn't occurred to me, or Steve, that he should accompany me, so I was alone in the waiting room. I hoped that I didn't appear as melancholy as some of the women; I didn't feel as sad as they looked, but I did feel crowded and wished I had more space.

The daily pricking and the sombre mood of the fertility clinic brought back feelings of when I was eleven trapped in a hospital bed, having my vital signs taken every fifteen minutes and blood measured daily. The veins on my hands and arms had become so black and blue from all the IV changes that they were no longer usable, and they had to surgically implant an IV in my upper chest, technically known as a central line, to administer my medications and fluids. I thought back to when I got my central line. It was the first of my surgeries. Although minor, with only a local anaesthetic, it had been performed in an operating room, and I had been taken in without my parents. I remember the doctor and nurses talking to me throughout the procedure, and also hearing the snip of the scissors as they cut my skin, and the wiggly sensation of the tube being inserted. I also recalled being petrified that if I moved I would cause myself great harm. I was very still and quiet, and kept my eyes closed until the doctor was done.

Often, when they looked for a good vein during the daily blood-taking at the fertility clinic I time-travelled back to when I was a child in hospital. I didn't want to, but my brain seemed determined to connect these events. My ovaries might not have been fertile ground, but the soil of my subconscious was rich with connections that left me feeling untethered. When I was young, I had to combat ulcerative colitis. Now, here I was again, at war with the body that had betrayed me. Back then, there was no jumping ship. I had no control of where or when they poked, prodded, inserted, measured and peered. I needed them to heal me so I could go home.

Now I had choices. I could decide to forgo the fertility clinic and just let Mother Nature take its course. Was that what I wanted to do? My fertility doctor had suggested that, even though my fallopian tubes were shown to be open, I might have a wall of scar tissue blocking the vicinity of the entrance. I had been examining, and breaking down, my emotional scar tissue for several years with Dr. Gaze. Now I had to investigate the physical remnants that were left behind in my abdomen. I assured myself that I had found my way over past medical hurdles, and this didn't feel insurmountable. My life wasn't in jeopardy, I had been doing some exploratory work in my conscious and subconscious, and now I'd be rooting around my reproductive area.

Chapter 21

Goldfinger

—∿—

"I never joke about my work, 007."   —Q, *Goldfinger*

After three months of cycle monitoring (blood-taking) Steve and I decided to step it up to the next level and do an artificial insemination, commonly referred to as a sperm wash. I hadn't been able to keep my childhood memories at bay during the daily needles, and the pre-sperm wash ultrasound added another dimension to my sojourn to darker times. The penis-shaped rod covered in a condom was inserted into my vagina to determine the placement of my ovaries and size of my eggs. This was not the first such measurement in the past few years.

I suppressed a lot of irritation as I lay quietly in the dark room, on the exam table, with my legs in the stirrups. The pain of the procedure was bearable, but the invasion of my body in the clinical setting still transported me back to a time of near death and emotional obliteration.

The technician wasn't supposed to tell me my results, but mine indicated that my ovaries were placed high and that she could see some bands of scar tissue. She said this so benignly as she adjusted the wand inside me for a better view. I was reminded of how I was spoken to when I was a child patient. I wanted to tell her to "fuck off" but remained polite and controlled. I was gripping the sides of the exam table, but trying to relax my pelvis. It was hard to control my emotions and the tension in my body.

After the ultrasound, I drove home in the glaring sun with tears streaming down my face. When I reached our apartment, I cried even harder remembering the awe I had felt as an adolescent returning to the very same neighbourhood. After I released my sorrow, things slowly became less surreal. The haziness evaporated, and anger bubbled to the surface. I was mad about the violation of my body.

Why couldn't the technician follow the rules and keep her mouth shut? I didn't want snippets of information to worry about. I was prepared to wait and discuss the results with the doctor. I disliked being thrown off guard with her unsolicited commentary. I was not one of those who tried and get information out of the people performing the test. I knew the drill. I had been raised to be, and was, polite. I was also introverted and shy by nature, so asking her to reserve her comments did not feel like an option to me. Therapy was helping me find my voice, but I was years away from feeling comfortable with speaking my mind. It's also hard to pipe up when you're experiencing the sensation of being outside your own skin.

A week later, my fertility doctor met with Mum and me to explain that she was concerned that my fallopian tubes may be closed due to past surgical scar tissue. She recommended a hysterosalpingogram, a more invasive x-ray, to have a better look. The exam was executed by Dr. Goldfinger. Can you imagine a better name for a gynecologist? James Bond fans will understand why, when I shook his hand, I was dying to introduce myself as Pussy Galore. Instead, I confirmed that I was Lindsay as I lay on the examining table.

The doctor then inserted a speculum into my vagina and cleaned my cervix. Next, a small tube called a cannula was placed into my cervix and my uterus was filled with iodine. The iodine contrasted with my fallopian tubes and uterus, giving the doctor a good picture in the x-ray. No 007 for me, I was the star of another type of film.

The hysterosalpingogram equipment was reminiscent of an unnerving diagnostic test I had endured in hospital. As a child, the x-ray was unlike anything I had experienced so far and my parents were not allowed to accompany me. I had to muster up my bravery knowing that I would be alone.

Back then, a flexible plastic tube, weighted with a sack of mercury, was inserted down my nose and throat to my stomach to help obtain a clear view of my intestines via ultrasound. I was aware that the doctors were still trying to establish what was causing my symptoms and this might help, but I was very troubled that the mercury sack might explode inside me. Could I be fatally poisoned? I was gently assisted in continually and carefully altering my body position on the gurney to accommodate a range of views on the technician's screen. I did exactly what I was told and was rewarded with "That's a good girl" "Good job" and "Not much longer." My steady round of Demerol shots left me feeling numb to what was going on with my body. I focused on my instructions and knew that tests didn't last forever so I should be done faster if I was compliant. I wanted to be back in the relative safety of my hospital room with my parents and nurses that I knew.

At Dr. Goldfinger's, I was still a very obedient and quiet patient. I was not physically numb, so when the iodine was shot through my reproductive area, because of my internal scar tissue and hence, tipped uterus, the hysterosalpingogram was painful; afterwards I felt faint and dead inside. Those feelings morphed into a detachment that took me out of my own body. I think I did that a lot as a kid too; it was often like I was watching myself on film and wasn't really there. I separated myself emotionally from the situation. As an adult, once I had privacy in the change room, I took some deep breaths, got dressed, and bought a juice at the café downstairs before I drove myself home. My movements were mechanical, but my mind couldn't keep everything tamped down. I was flooded with memories of the terror I felt when I had been taken for my first surgery and was wheeled away from my family to the operating room.

Days later, reviewing my hysterosalpingogram results, my fertility doctor explained to me that my fallopian tubes were open, but scar tissue was making it hard for the sperm to get to the tubes. This, coupled with the fact that I had high placed ovaries meant that in vitro fertilization might not be a plausible option. I had been considering it even although I knew it meant drugs; close cycle monitoring and $8,000. Although it was a lot of money, I figured it would be worth it. Steve always grew quiet when we discussed our fertility; he seemed resentful of the potential cost, but let me grab the reins for this ride. Thus far, money hadn't been able to rid me of my ileostomy, or of colitis, so if we could buy something to help our sperm and eggs meet, then I figured we should try it. If we could purchase our way to a family, then it was money well spent. When we learned that in vitro might not work, we immediately dismissed the idea. It had sounded like the hormone injections would put my body through a lot of stress anyway, so there was a part of me that was relieved.

Steve and I were at a crossroads with our fertility options, and he was leaving it up to me to decide what path to take. I wanted to be a mother and he wanted me to have what I wanted. He told me he would be happy with or without children, as long as he had me. I realize now that parenthood is a partnership, so at the time I felt uncomfortable being in charge of our future family; but I was so used to being perceived as strong that I let him off the hook.

I had sometimes wondered if my body was meant to have babies with an abdomen that had already been through so much. I knew my parents worried about the strain that a pregnancy would have on my body. I had the same anxieties. I didn't openly discuss these gnawing doubts with anyone for the fear that I would somehow jinx my ability to have a baby. It was not until I talked to my "stump surgeon" that I finally got the truth. I told her that I was going to start trying to conceive. She said, "Well, there is so much technology these days, it may take a while, but *should* be possible."

And suddenly I knew—all those surgeries had affected my reproductive organs. Pregnancy was not a given, it was actually very unlikely.

I had been thinking this for years. It made sense. How could it be possible to slice someone up repeatedly, move things around and not have some long-term internal repercussions that affect the ability to reproduce? In my mind, I went further and wondered if the many anaesthetics, medications and traumatic recovery periods could have further weakened and permanently damaged my immune system.

As a youngster, my doctor visits had been much simpler and I had known my parents would take care of me so I didn't have to worry too much about the details. All I had wanted was to get better and go home. But now that I was an adult, it wasn't so simple. I was responsible for my own health decisions. I could no longer be passive; I had to weigh risks and benefits and think things through for myself. It took some getting used to and was daunting and empowering at the same time.

—⁊⁊—

There had been seven surgeries between when I was eleven years old and when I started to pursue fertility options, most of them when I was an adolescent. I was now practiced at talking through my medical history in therapy. I was exploring things about myself, and this organically drew me back to something I had always enjoyed, writing. A friend recently shared a quote from my Grade 6 yearbook that states, "I like spelling and creative movement."

After I graduated with a Bachelor of Science, I went back to school, while working full time at Sick Kids, and took two university English classes, receiving straight A's. I loved those courses. I must have—the classroom was a fifty-minute drive from my house. I'm nervous driving at night and left class with the moon shining down on me from the pitch-black sky. I would fall into bed around 11 pm and was ready to go at my desk by 8 am the next morning.

I enjoyed homework and started to regularly and enthusiastically participate in class. That was a first for me, and it felt so good. I was like a baby chick, pecking my way out of her egg. Investigating my new perspectives was invigorating. My teacher was fantastic. Her name was Rita Bode and I will never forget how she opened my eyes to the joy of learning.

Several years later, I followed those English courses with a night class in creative writing at Ryerson, a university in Toronto, close to where I worked and lived. As I was approaching my 32nd birthday and embarking on fertility treatments I wrote a personal piece called "Images of War" for an assignment. It was after writing this that my instructor encouraged me to write more. She suggested that my thoughts might prove useful to others going through traumatic situations. I took her comments to heart and kept writing. It started out as therapeutic and somehow started to take the shape of a memoir, or more specifically, it became the inspiration behind the start of this book.

Chapter 22

What's next?

—∞—

"I have a thing about angels. I believe in them. I feel like I have a guardian angel. I think everyone has one." —Sheryl Lee

It was the spring of 2001, and I had been experiencing weakness and numbness in my right hand and was sleeping a lot more than usual after work and on the weekends. I questioned whether I was depressed about not being able to become pregnant, but after several years of talking therapy, I knew that having occasional feelings of sadness didn't necessarily mean I was depressed. Anyway, depression wouldn't explain my hand. A month later, I went to the doctor. My neck was x-rayed because she thought the tingling was the result of some nerve damage in that area of my body. The x-rays showed two small bone spurs in the left side of my neck. I was diagnosed with a pinched nerve in my neck and prescribed physio and massage therapy.

The numbness persisted throughout the summer and I began to frequently drop things. At work, files seemed to carelessly slip out of my hand; I took care not to lift anything heavy in case I further damaged my neck.

Two years prior, Steve and I had bought a cottage with my mum. She had always wanted a summer place outside the city, and so had we. By sharing the cost of the cottage, it became affordable. I loved our bungalow on the lake and we vacationed there every summer as we fixed it up. Steve left the decorating up to me and Mum. He and his father installed a new kitchen, with white wood shaker-style cabinets, royal blue counter tops and a backsplash with handcrafted, white subway tiles. When you stood at the kitchen sink you had a view of the lake. We painted the new drywall in the living area "light-house yellow," white-washed the ceiling, and installed pale laminate wood floors. Mum was working on weekends at a furniture store, so we bought some good quality, comfy sofas covered in blue and white striped cotton slip covers.

I loved the cheery and relaxed aesthetic of the cottage surrounded by trees and the lake. We continued to invite guests each weekend to our newly purchased and renovated summer retreat, and I slowly began to dread it. I was regularly experiencing fatigue and the cottage represented continual work. On Monday mornings I would feel exhausted instead of rejuvenated.

While vacationing at our cottage in July, I decided to step up the pace of my usual walk along the dirt country road and went for a short jog. Mid route, my right leg inexplicably began to drag and, not knowing what was happening, I decided to turn back and walk the remainder of the way home. I couldn't make my leg move properly. It didn't feel like it belonged to me. Someone, or something else, was controlling it.

In shock, the thought that kept itself in the front of my mind was, "Don't let the neighbours see." I didn't know what was going on, but I was used to my health issues being undercover and didn't feel like sharing my worries. Also, denial is a very strange thing; it can trick our brain into thinking useless thoughts when fear strikes.

When I got home, I told Steve what had happened and retreated to the cocoon of our bed for a nap, reasoning that, while I surrounded myself in our cozy duvet and shut my eyes, my leg would recover and the increased tingling in my right hand would stop. I instinctively knew I needed to rest and take care of myself, but I had the feeling my husband thought I was being lazy. Steve was unconvinced that there was anything wrong with me. I felt angry and misunderstood when he clearly thought I was trying to shirk work that needed done around the cottage. The truth was I found it very difficult to hold a paintbrush, broom or rake for any extended period of time, and my hand became numb and claw-like when I tried.

At thirty-one, I put my symptoms down to internal war wounds and age, and that was the story I was trying to stick to. But I was a fit, non-smoking, well-nourished young woman unable to take a leisurely jog, let alone brush her teeth without working hard to hold onto the tooth brush—what the hell was happening to me? I kept telling myself that I wasn't a teenager anymore and, since my surgery three years prior, my body hadn't been the same, but I was having a hard time kidding myself. The educated, rational me wasn't buying what I was desperately trying to sell, so you can imagine what the paranoid me was speculating.

That evening, although my hand was still weak, my leg seemed to work normally, but I was sufficiently worried to make an appointment with my doctor. I was scared, but I wanted to know what was going on with my body. The feelings of confusion and fear were reminiscent of years earlier when I had been very ill, didn't know what was wrong, and ended up with a bag on my stomach. I knew how mysterious illnesses could turn out, and was secretly terrified.

Outwardly to my family, I tried to convey an optimism that wasn't really there. I don't think I even talked about my symptoms with my friends or colleagues. I discussed my anxieties with Dr. Gaze because my years of experience with bowel disease had taught me to listen to my body. I sensed it was betraying me again and I had something more than a pinched nerve. After seven years of psychotherapy, I had the skills to talk about my emotions, not suppress them. I knew I was scared, but didn't want to concern those who loved me.

I meditated when I had moments to myself, fondly remembering my summers in Vermont. I longed for my aunt. I missed the companionship of the horses, and that they expected so little of me for the immense pleasure they gave.

—〰—

After the dragging leg incident at the cottage, my family doctor sent me to a neurologist in her building. Upon entering her office, I immediately noticed the walls were covered in sports memorabilia, specifically baseball. I barely followed sports, and, at the time, found baseball particularly boring. Steve's family bonded over sports, but I always zoned out of the conversations. Maybe I should have listened so I'd have something in common with this doctor. It can be hard to connect with physicians, but I wanted to be seen as human, not just a case number. That didn't happen. Without suggesting any possible causes of my symptoms, I was given a requisition for an MRI of my neck and brain. I asked her what might explain my numbness. She responded cryptically, "It could be as simple as a slipped disk."

I didn't think so, and I could tell by the way she delivered that unconvincing line, that she didn't either. After my appointment, on the way home in the car, Mum and I were quiet. I had talked to the doctor alone. I thought that was how I should act as a grown-up.

As we drove away from the medical building, my mother asked me what the doctor had said. I recounted the doctor's indistinct remarks, but didn't have much to add because I hadn't probed further. I could tell that Mum was frustrated that I hadn't asked more questions, but she likely realized I wasn't ready to know too much. Not from a doctor anyway. I went about gathering some information on my own, and brought my mum into all of my next neurologist appointments.

I realized after that first visit that I should have someone accompany me to the doctor, even if they just listened. I needed another set of ears because it was easy to get overwhelmed by the information coming at me, especially if it was upsetting. Most brains can only process, and hold on to, a certain amount of information. I began asking Mum to take notes at scheduled visits with my new doctors. That way, I could focus on listening, without stressing about retaining the information. She and I would both ask questions.

One night I was having dinner with Steve and Courtenay. My right hand had been very tired that day so we had a laugh about "the claw" as I carefully picked up my wine glass. I needed a sense of humour, but what I was thinking wasn't funny. I calmly shared that I thought I might have MS. My husband looked irritated and gave me a sideways glance while bluntly stating, "You don't have MS."

Court didn't say anything. I have often thought that one of the worst punishments in life I could receive would be something happening to my sister. Our relationship is sometimes complicated, but the love is not. I knew that the possibility of me having MS was not crazy to her, just exceedingly sorrowful.

At dinner I went on to substantiate my self-diagnosis. I related the fact that my symptoms were consistent with MS. I explained that, after browsing a few websites, I determined I was a textbook case study of the disease. I was a woman in my thirties, of northern European descent with fatigue, numbness, weakness, and clumsiness in her hand and leg. Were the doctors not saying this aloud to me because I also had a stiff neck? Half the population has problems with their neck.

At this point, the person who had been most candid with regards to my symptoms was my massage therapist Diana. I liked her—she had a new-age, hippy kind of vibe, and would have fit in well in California. Her office was a room in her apartment and was decorated with crystal rocks, blankets and wind chimes; the back ground noise of our sessions was a recording of the ocean. Her yellow Labrador Retriever came and went out of the treatment room. I trusted Diana and asked her to tell me what she thought was causing my symptoms. I beseeched her to be straightforward with her reply. She had been treating me for a few months, since my hand had become numb and weak, and Diana and I seemed to share an understanding. I had cried during her first treatment. As she released my tension with her massage skills, she kept a flow of conversation going.

During one visit I began to talk to her about my dad's illness the previous summer and Aunt Jill's death nine years earlier. I was getting teary as I talked about my dad's recent recovery from an aneurism when Diana asked me "Lindsay, do you have a personal angel?"

That concept was new to me, but I didn't hesitate with my reply, "My parents are my angels on the ground."

I was lying on my front and Diana waited as I adjusted myself on the table to better fit my face in the hole of the headspace. Once comfortable, I continued, "I'm not religious, so I have kind of made up my own heaven. My own views on life after death usually involve a spiritual world where the few people I have lost are looking down on their loved ones and sending some sort of energy."

"Hmmm, that sounds nice." Diana said, sincerely.

I felt mildly embarrassed so I explained "I know that my beliefs are flimsy, but it has helped me cope. I often feel my Aunt Jill's presence when I'm going through hard times. I feel like she is watching out for me. I guess that makes her my angel up there."

I moved my wrists around as best as I could under the sheet to indicate the ceiling, or sky.

Diana continued to work her hands gently on my neck and asked me, "She was obviously very special to you. Do you feel her spirit often?"

A tear dripped on the floor as I said, "Yes, especially when I'm really happy or sad; like when my parents separated while Courtenay was travelling abroad, when I was getting my hair done on my wedding day, when I suntanned on the black pebble beach with my girlfriends in Santorini, or when I'm riding a horse through the trails in Vermont."

Diana replied, "Her spirit sounds strong; it lives within you."

And, as if on cue, Diana's cat crept into the room and circled under the massage table. She leapt up on the neighbouring chair and made herself comfortable on my folded clothes.

I giggled and Diana asked "Do you mind?"

"Not in the least, she'll keep my clothes warm."

I really felt Diana understood when she stated simply "You are lucky to have such a supportive family."

I smiled as I replied, "I know it. They are my biggest blessing. We have always been there for each other, especially during health challenges. My mum and dad are split but she was still there every day for him while he recovered from his aneurism last year."

Diana seemed genuinely impressed when she remarked "That is rare."

"It is, but we come together when we need to. Dad flew to LA to be by his sister's side when she was battling cancer and she flew to mine when I was fighting ulcerative colitis. They both often took transatlantic flights when Grandpa was sick. I even spent a week with my aunt in California when she was battling cancer because I wanted to be close to her."

I didn't want to sob so I continued my thoughts privately. As much as I needed to be with her, my Aunt Jill had wanted me there. There was no doubt in my mind that our love was mutual and that she needed me too.

Diana's angel inquiry fit very well with my version of the after world. During our session, Diana tapped into my need for Aunt Jill. My parents had already been through so much pain with me. I wished she were there to help share their burden. She had broadened the scope of support when I was a child. I needed the safety net of my family because I intuitively knew that I did not have a slipped disk, and I was well past the point of thinking that bad things would not happen to me. I also knew that my family is strong, but who wants to be the reason for bad news?

Diana's massages felt good and relaxed me but they didn't fix the weakness and tingling in my limbs. I thought that she was smart and honest so I wanted to get her opinion on my condition. I waited until I was paying the bill to ask. I was standing up and dressed—less vulnerable. "What do you think is happening here? I don't think I have a slipped disk. It doesn't make sense to me. Why am I so tired? And please don't sugar coat your reply. Tell me what you really think. I'm not a china doll, I won't break."

Diana looked me straight in the eye and said, "You're right, it doesn't make sense. Your leg and hand wouldn't likely be affected the way they are presenting together. My best guess is that you have MS or a brain tumour."

I said, "My bets are on MS." It felt like a relief to say it out loud and have it validated.

Diana confirmed what had been swimming in my head for weeks. A slipped disk didn't make sense because of the dragging leg. Although terrified, it felt like a compliment being treated as an intelligent human being. It made me feel less of a loony for fearing the worst. I am not a fatalist, but a realist, and I don't appreciate doctors tiptoeing around me.

Chapter 23

Interferon interference

—⚹—

"Carpenter ants are a widespread nuisance and major cause of structural damage." —Wikipedia

I needed Dr. Gaze again. After about six years of seeing her, in 2000, when I was thirty-one, I had decided to end therapy. We had accomplished a lot and I no longer felt weighted down by old trauma and sadness. However, when I started experiencing MS symptoms, I worried and wanted to ensure that I had some trusted emotional support in place for when I was diagnosed with *something* even though I didn't know what yet. I explained this as I asked Dr. Gaze to resume our appointments. I told her, "I think something is coming down the pipe medically for me. I believe there is something wrong neurologically."

I knew. I could feel it in my body. I understood my mechanics all too well, and knew that I wasn't a car that needed a quick tire replacement, my motor was breaking down. I was aware of how lonely and scared compromised health could make me feel, and so I prepared to face my newest challenge. I had no problem securing a weekly appointment again. Dr. Gaze knew I wouldn't ask unless I needed it.

During this time, I received my MRI results and was referred to an orthopedic surgeon regarding my neck. At the appointment he told me and my mum "It's nice to meet you, but I'm not sure why you were referred to me. I don't think you are a candidate for surgery."

That was good news, but I had been surprised that I might need surgery, and he wasn't smiling so I continued listening before I celebrated too much.

"If I operated on the deterioration of your neck, it might leave you unable to turn your head, and I don't think you need to consider this, judging by your MRI."

Mum and I were stunned. An immobile neck? That outcome had never been on my radar. I was very glad he didn't think I needed that operation. I asked him about what the MRI had shown in my brain.

His response was "The MRI was only of your neck."

I kept my cool, but was frustrated. I had been told my neck *and* brain were being scanned. I felt like valuable time had been wasted and was upset that I still didn't have a diagnosis. Unfortunately, due to some error, the MRI was only performed on my neck, the brain was left out. The surgeon suggested I should have another MRI, this time, of my brain. Instead of him ordering it, he referred me to a colleague of his, a neurologist, Dr. Smith.

We left the office deflated, but I was full of purpose. I wanted answers. We walked across the hall to make an appointment with the neurologist.

A few weeks later, Mum and I sat opposite Dr. Smith as he asked me about my symptoms and performed an in-office exam. I told him I had been taking Tylenol for the tingles in my hand. He raised an eyebrow and asked "How's that been going for you?"

I sheepishly replied, "It hasn't helped."

He smiled kindly, but was very matter of fact when he told me "I would be shocked if you don't have MS. I'm going to order an MRI of your brain. Sometimes MS can take a while to present itself in an MRI, so if your brain comes back clear, we'll do another one in six months."

Mum and I were silent so he continued "Sometimes the spots on the brain take a while to show even if the disease is present."

I don't remember how we wrapped up the appointment, but I received the requisition for an MRI and we were solemn as we walked to the car. Mum was downcast, but I was seething with rage. Even before I had an MRI of my brain, Dr. Smith was so matter-of-fact about me probably having MS; it was so much more to me. If he had loaded that sentence into an arrow, and shot it from a taut bow,

I had a feeling it was a bull's eye shot. It seemed easy to say, but it was counter intuitive to me to search for, and chase a diagnosis that I didn't want.

I kept it together during the appointment, but afterwards I released a barrage of curses and then, exhausted, cried in the car while Mum drove me back to work. I was so tired of being in coping mode that I yearned to creep into a cave and disappear for a few months. Hibernating in the dark held momentary appeal. I was mad that I had to wait and see, and deal with the unknown. Mum suggested not being strong and to crawl into bed to just feel sad and sleep. This is her way and is very rarely mine. Mum can sometimes shut down. Depression can get the better of her and it is not easy to watch. It took me and my sister a long time to understand that although our mother intellectually knows what to do to help herself, sometimes she simply can't do it. She will spend a few days mostly in bed, and then rally. We are wired differently that way. While I can appreciate the sheer relief of avoidance and how it can help for an hour or two, I feel stronger if I confront my pain head on and dive into my emotional whirlpool, usually confident that I will emerge swimming. It's the only way I don't drown.

After six weeks of waiting for my second round of MRI results, I got the call from my neurologist, Dr. Smith. I was at my desk in the accounting department of a large finance company, and saw "Smith" flash on my phone's call display. My coworkers sat near me, but were engrossed in their work. Still, I looked around tentatively as I lifted the handset. My voice was steady but my hand was trembling as I answered.

"Hello, Lindsay speaking."

"Hi Lindsay, it's Dr. Smith."

The phone's technology had already given him away, but I didn't let on as I replied, "Oh, hi, Dr. Smith, how are you?"

"Well, I'm ok," he responded, "but I got your MRI results back and they confirmed you have MS."

My body flipped the off switch and I felt weak and powerless as I withered in my seat. My voice was as small as I felt, but I managed squeak out, "Ok."

The other end of the phone continued, "I did try and prepare you on your last visit."

Ever polite, I confirmed what he said. "Oh, yes, you did, thanks."

Dr. Smith continued, "You have relapsing-remitting MS. I think I explained the different types of the disease when you were last in my office."

This was true, but now that I actually had the dreaded disease, I knew I needed to pay close attention. I started taking some point form notes on the yellow post-it notes on my desk. I would stick them to the inside of my purse later. I wrote down as much as I could.

"RRMS presents as unpredictable, but clearly defined relapses," he said. "We also call them flare-ups, attacks or exacerbations. New symptoms may appear during these attacks, or existing ones get worse. In the period between relapses, usually a full recovery is made, or a nearly complete recovery to like before the relapse."

I needed to hear more about the remissions, so I jumped in. "So, I'm in a relapse right now with my draggy leg and weak hand, how will I know when I remit?"

Dr. Smith patiently replied, "Your symptoms will go away. It can take days or months. When the symptoms first start you can take prednisone to possibly speed up recovery. You have been in this relapse too long for that to be effective now."

I shivered, and had goose bumps, it was all so cold and clinical. I needed some hope, so I continued with remission questions. "So, you think I will remit from this relapse?"

Maybe he sensed my fear because his voice was gentle as he replied, "Yes, I do, Lindsay. Your MRI showed only white plaques in your brain. This means the disease is active, but black plaques indicate permanent damage and you don't have any of those."

I didn't ask when my spots might become black. I didn't want to know.

With excellent timing, Dr. Smith threw me a life preserver. "The good news is there are disease-modifying therapies that are available to help minimize the effects of the disease. These drugs are also called immunomodulatory therapies. Their goal is to reduce relapses and slow disease progression. They work by targeting some aspect of the inflammatory process."

My notes read "drug treatments." I knew the answer, but I asked anyway, "The drugs don't cure MS, right?"

He calmy stated "No, their goal is to reduce relapses and that reduces disease progression. They work by targeting some aspect of the inflammatory process. Three of the drugs are interferons; Avonex, Betaseron and Rebif. The fourth is Copaxone, a synthetic protein. All four treatments are given by self-injection."

I silently thought, needles . . . great.

Dr. Smith began wrapping things up, "Come by my office this week to pick up the reading materials I have on MS and the treatment options. You can decide what is the best choice for you."

That seemed like a big decision for me to make. I didn't ask, but shouldn't he tell me what to do? He gave me some direction when he said "The faster you start taking treatment the better. Less relapses are a good thing."

I felt an urgency to get going and to get off the phone so I said "I'll come by tomorrow. Is there a treatment that you think is best?"

Staying on the fence, Dr. Smith replied "It really is a personal preference. Do you have health insurance?"

Thankfully, I could reply "Yes."

"Ok, good. The drugs are very expensive. Rebif has slightly better relapse rates, but it's also the most expensive."

I hadn't even waded into the topic of potential side effects of the medications or how I would inject them. I was done. My brain couldn't upload any more information. Words were becoming vocal swirls. I wish it had been like looking through my childhood kaleidoscope, but it was more akin to being a house in a tropical storm, without hurricane shutters in place. I couldn't listen to the words;

they were too fast and swerving past the processing centre in my brain. My now confirmed diseased brain.

Like a programmed robot, I said "Thank you, once I have read everything, I'll let you know if I have any questions."

"Sounds like a plan, Lindsay. Bye."

"Bye, Dr. Smith, thank you."

Another day at the office for my doctor. The same couldn't be said for me; it was official—I now had MS.

All the sounds around me echoed. The conversations in neighbouring cubicles sounded distant. The beige walls, black office chairs, fluorescent lighting and grey industrial carpet never seemed so ugly before; my co-workers always brightened how I perceived things. Now my office friends, and the personal memorabilia on their desks, shrank into the background, and the office lost its warmth.

I walked slowly, in a fog, to a small, bare and vacant private meeting room that was usually reserved for the auditors, and called my husband at his office. I stiffly relayed the news to him, but I could feel my protective film disintegrating as my tears began to flow, the salty droplets puckering my shield. Steve listened and said "I'm leaving work, we need to go home. Are you ok to get to your mum's house? I parked there today. Meet me there and we'll get home. I love you."

That sounded like a good plan, so I replied, "I love you too, I'll see you at Mum's."

I desperately needed to go home and talk to my trusted defenders, my family. After I hung up, I blotted my eyes, readjusted my posture, and strode back to my desk. I still looked composed, and wanted to get out of the office before that façade was too difficult to maintain. I fired off an email to my boss telling him my diagnosis, that I was going home, and that I'd see him the next day.

I couldn't bear to be on the busy subway, surrounded by strangers; I took a cab the short distance to my mum's house. I let myself in, left the door unlocked for Steve and went upstairs to find Mum in her bedroom. She knew something was wrong because I didn't usually pop in during a work day. I could see the worry on her face so I quickly told her why I was there. "Mum, I heard from Dr. Smith and I have MS."

We crawled into her unmade bed as we waited for Steve to arrive. Mum got me an extra blanket and I warmed up my frigid feet on her warm ones. My mother had been expecting the news, but there was always a vestige of hope that there was a less drastic explanation for what was happening to me. Hope now bulldozed, we retreated under the covers and, as I saw my mum's face crumple in suppressed grief, I told her to cry and I held her, as she has held me often in the past, and she let her body give way to the sorrow. There would be plenty of moments for us to buck each other up, now was the time to get through the shock and sadness. Just being with her helped me.

We laid in her king-sized bed and held each other, and I felt comforted by her presence and the familiar surroundings. The bookshelves were filled with well-known books that were a sort of buttress for my anguish, many of which I had read, including Aunt Jill's memoirs. Her works *Life Wish* and *Life Lines* were reminders that this was life: my life. I felt spent but safe and, by the time Steve arrived, I was nestled under a fuzzy blanket gathering my thoughts. Once we collected ourselves, I telephoned Dad and Courtenay. A few hours later, when I was home, I reached out to a handful of my close girlfriends.

My stage of shock wasn't the textbook experience I had read about on the Internet. *Why me?* was not part of the equation. I mean really, why not me? I had emotional resources from my past experiences and therapy that a lot of newly diagnosed people would not. So did my family. I felt a weird mixture of numbness and motivation. I was motivated by fear to fight the disease, but felt distanced again, like I was watching myself in a movie.

It was surreal, even as I dove into figuring out my new reality. For the first week or two after my diagnosis, I would search the Internet several times a day at work, sometimes only looking at The MS Society of Canada website for two minutes. I would log on again an hour later to do the same thing. I needed to continually present myself with information to help work through the shock.

I knew I had one auto immune disease, ulcerative colitis, and I remembered, at my pre-MS diagnosis appointments, Dr. Smith had told me that it is not uncommon for people to end up with another. That had been hard to hear so I hadn't pursued that information. But I wanted to know more about MS and as I did my research, I learned that MS is thought to be an autoimmune disease of the central nervous system (brain and spinal cord). The disease attacks myelin, the protective covering of the nerves, causing inflammation and often damaging the myelin. Myelin is necessary for the transmission of nerve impulses through nerve fibres. If damage to myelin is slight, nerve impulses travel with minor interruptions; however, if damage is heavy and if scar tissue replaces the myelin, nerve impulses may be completely disrupted, and the nerve fibres themselves can be damaged.

I had been diagnosed because of numbness and weakness in my hand and leg. As I researched the disease, the list of unpredictable symptoms was terrifying. The words floated from the screen into my brain and I focused on not shutting down so they could make their way to my processing centre. I learned that not all people with MS experience all the possible symptoms, and the severity of the disease can vary greatly between patients. Some people with MS have very few symptoms, and a few actually have none. It's rare, but it happens. Still, the list of symptoms was long and overwhelming. The fact that they can crop up out of the blue was especially frightening. The most common symptoms seemed to be fatigue, numbness and tingling, weakness, cognitive impairment, spasticity, optic neuritis (which may cause blindness), bladder and bowel dysfunction, difficulty with speech and swallowing, mood swings, sexual dysfunction, tremors, dry mouth, and depression. Depression? No kidding. I found that easy to understand after reading the list.

I wanted to stay positive; I decided to gather an arsenal of information to help me feel informed in combating the disease. I read about the interferon drugs that my doctor had suggested, and about food and fitness choices I could make to possibly help control symptoms. I also investigated dietary supplements and made an appointment with the naturopath at my masseuse Diana's new clinic. I immediately decided to choose one of the three interferon treatments offered at the time. I chose the drug that had slightly better statistics at controlling relapses than the others, which would hopefully slow disease progression. Luckily, with my health insurance, I didn't have to factor cost into my decisions.

I decided to start taking Rebif as soon as possible. Rebif is considered an immunosuppressant because it is thought to work by stopping the immune system from attacking the myelin sheath. I was working in the pilot mode of shock as I scheduled an appointment with a nurse to come and teach me to inject myself with Rebif. I had endured so many needles as a kid that what they represented hurt more than the actual prick. They reminded me of pain and imminent death. I had to get over that in a hurry.

My MS diagnosis did not surprise me; Dr. Smith had all but told me I had MS without seeing any MRI results. That, along with my own intuition and research, had prepared me for the truth. Still, until they'd had a look in my brain, and I actually had my results, I had secretly clung to the very flimsy chance that there was a less severe reason for my symptoms. A few summers earlier I had been hiking with Su through the hills in L.A. and we talked about her fears for the future, and specifically, the hereditary nature of breast cancer. Long before Angelina Jolie made the notion mainstream, Su had considered having her breasts removed as a preventative measure. The hot August California sun was pounding down on us when I suggested that that might be drastic. She countered by saying, "Well, you're in the clear; you've already gone through all your stuff years ago." How interesting that she felt that made me exempt from more disease.

We sat down in the dusty dirt to watch a mama coyote and her babies in the distance; I felt grounded to the earth, and had the sense that the sun was baking my response as the words hit the air. I responded, saying, "I wish that was true, but there's no guy in the sky rationing out disease, ill health or fortune."

Walking home, we recalled how Su gave me the nickname Gutsy when we were kids. I never asked her why until that day. She explained her admiration for how I was always up for an adventure and that I endured my surgeries with positivity. She thought I had tremendous guts. The irony of my disease being in my stomach made us laugh. Her words from two years prior were sounding in my ears when I thought of now having bowel disease, an ileostomy and MS by the time I was thirty-two. What would be next? And who's still testing my gutsiness? I think I passed long ago.

I had learned copious amounts about myself by reliving and discussing childhood pain, and those insights stood me in good stead while dealing with my MS diagnosis. A friend suggested that I must be very bitter about what has happened in my life; the ileostomy, the fertility issues and then MS. My biggest fear is bitterness; bitter people are so depleting to be around. I believe that bitterness not only infects those at the receiving end, but also is poisonous for those harbouring the resentment. I have an image of bitterness being like carpenter ants that slowly eat away and erode good, strong, pure wood. The destruction is devastating.

Chapter 24

Spirit

—∿—

"The secret of change is to focus all of your energy, not on fighting the old, but on building the new." —Socrates

I might have been afraid of bitterness, but I was still mad about my newfound neurological companion, MS. It had taken two neurologists and several months to be diagnosed. I needed to wrap my head around the fact that my right hand might never be the same and that the "I can hardly move" fatigue could be a regular part of my life. Taking a nap didn't alleviate the exhaustion. That was the relatively easy part; these symptoms would come and go in "attacks" or "relapses" with new conditions cropping up without warning. Suddenly my upper lip would be numb and my smile crooked. My grin was off balance and so was I. I would go to bed and feel fine, and wake up to pins and needles in my hand, feet or face. Sometimes it would last for a few hours, sometimes days. The leg and hand weakness had been coming and going for months.

It was hard to understand, and explain to others, that MS fatigue was overwhelming and wasn't fixed by rest. There was a new war being waged in my body, but there was no clear route to peace. My fear was that there would never be peace, as I knew it, again. You couldn't just cut out the enemy with a scalpel. The counterattack was hard to plan. Unlike my childhood experience, the doctors weren't the only ones in charge. Furthermore, they were talking directly to me, not my parents. I thought I had the fortitude to face what lay ahead, but I needed to keep gathering information because I was the general heading up this army. Invisibility was not an option.

I had been told over and over by Mum, Dad and Aunt Jill that I was strong like my Grandpa Jack. He had one health problem after another but never appeared to lose his unwavering will to live. First, at age fifty old he was hit by a heart attack, then a triple bypass, then Crohn's disease resulting in a colostomy, then a stroke, and then another stroke. Life chipped away at him, but somehow, through sheer stubbornness, he would manage to apply some putty to the cracks and keep standing. His last stroke took away his ability to talk so he could not verbally express his deepest thoughts and emotions. He coped with that until he lost his daughter, my aunt Jill. After her death, he let his walls crumble and turn to dust.

I mostly felt proud when my family compared me to Grandpa because he always seemed strong and resilient. He charged through all his health trials. He enjoyed family outings, travel, card games, and, even without the use of his spoken and written words, usually somehow got us to understand his basic needs and wishes. He could hear

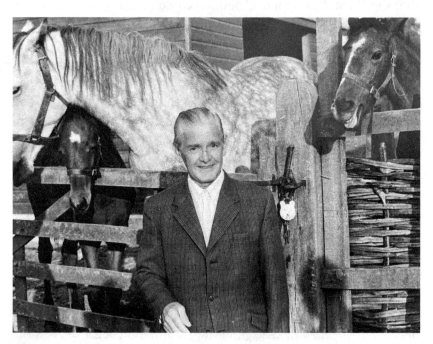

Grandpa Ireland before his stroke. He loved horses too.

the words he wanted to say in his head, but they came out of his mouth as "lo, de do, de do, lo, lo, lo." He expressed his frustration with one of the only phrases he had access to, "Fuffin' hell!" Depending on his delivery, this was either hilarious or heart breaking. When he wanted to add some levity to a situation, he'd rally us to sing with him, and we'd happily belt out "Daisy, Daisy." He still knew all the words to that one.

Upon reflection with Dr. Gaze, I realized that Grandpa having a colostomy had been another thing that affected the way I perceived my ileostomy. I thought of my bag as an old man's affliction. I knew that a lot of people thought ostomies were for the elderly. Many times, in my youth, health care workers, or the staff at the surgical supply store where I bought my ostomy supplies, expressed surprise that I had a bag because "I was so young." It reinforced my desire to keep my bag a secret. I didn't want to be thought of in the same category as old men. I wanted to be a normal young girl.

When I had my ostomy surgeries, and later found out I had MS, I was much younger than when Grandpa had his first heart attack, but with this new diagnosis, I sensed that my healthy outer layer of cement was slowly and methodically being eroded. Would the foundation begin to crumble? I was determined not to let that happen; I had too much to do.

I thought of Aunt Jill and how, if she were still here, what she would have said to me. In my mind I could hear her voice breaking as she told me everything was going to be all right, that it's okay to cry, and I am strong. That we would get through it like everything else. The problem with my imagined script was that the last statement was untrue. She didn't get through it. She fought and lost.

I had to keep reminding myself that MS wouldn't kill me. Instead of thoughts of dying, I became obsessed with the fear of ending up crippled. Every time I saw someone in a wheelchair, I wondered if they had MS—especially if they were female—even more so, if they were young. Who am I kidding? Every wheelchair screamed MS to me. It was just deafening if they were my age and gender. The noise was electric in my brain. My thoughts were crippling, never mind the disease.

I tried to push morbid ideas from my mind, but my defenses were down. I hadn't been expecting another major disease so soon. I needed to feel empowered and not so scared. That fortitude my family was always talking about felt as essential as the air that I breathed. Aunt Jill had taught me about the benefits of alternative medicine, and my family believed in these too. They supported the idea of me researching and trying new ways to better my health. I knew that there must be some non-traditional approaches that I could try. This is where the Internet came in handy. I searched it prudently, bypassing sites that hawked "miracle pills." Every reputable site listed yoga and swimming as beneficial forms of exercise for MS patients. Madonna and other movie stars had recently helped make yoga mainstream and fashionable, so I had been thinking about trying it for several years, and now had an excellent reason to sign up for a session. There's nothing like a firm diagnosis of a neurological disease to get you in gear. Registering for a class and buying a yoga mat was the first step. I was doing something besides living in dread of losing the ability to walk.

At my first yoga class, once everyone was on their downward dog pose, the instructor came over to introduce herself and ask me about myself. While inverted, I explained that an MS diagnosis had brought me to the practice of yoga. She crouched down as she replied, "The brain can be retrained; I'm so glad you are here."

I liked that; a lot. Being open about MS felt easy, it was so different than how I felt about my ostomy. I didn't feel any shame. It made it easier to garner bits of support and encouragement from outside my inner circle.

The first yoga lesson was a bit advanced, but not frustratingly so; I tried again. And again. And again. Each time I unrolled my pink yoga mat I felt like I was part of something bigger. The inclusive power of the collective "Ommmmmm," to begin and end each class felt like a tribal call for calm and health.

When we did the deep breathing to start the class, my favourite instructor told us to breathe in the positive energy and breathe out the negative. I took it a step further and breathed out the bad MS cells and inhaled healthy cells. I pushed out the nasty MS karma, and sucked in strength and vitality, exhaled the spots on my brain, making the space in my head clear again. If I could have done an MRI right there and then I would have put big money on the fact that the lesions had disappeared.

I experienced the sensation of my brain flooding with the bright white healing light that Aunt Jill had channelled through meditation and crystals. She would have been proud. My mum had touted the benefits of deep breathing when I was in hospital as a child. She had led me through the very breathing exercises that I was now doing in yoga classes about twenty years later. When I told Mum about the yoga and the breathing, she proudly told me that her yoga instructor in the 70s had used her as an example to the class about how to employ yogic breath. I felt exceptionally lucky to have had two broad-minded, forward-thinking women influencing the way I viewed the world.

Like therapy, Steve thought yoga, crystals and meditation were for flaky types of people. He had never met my aunt, but she was not flaky. She did chemotherapy and supplemented her fight against cancer with these other less toxic, self-help treatments. I considered her methods resourceful and thoughtful. Grandpa had shown us what a strong will could achieve. I never questioned the benefits of alternative therapies because I knew they gave hope and hope is a very powerful thing. I needed hope and continued to use non-traditional treatments in addition to the medically approved drug, Rebif.

Chapter 25

9/11

"What separates us from the animals, what separates us from the chaos, is our ability to mourn people we have never met."   —David Levithan

Three weeks after my MS diagnosis, Steve was fired from his job. He had been recruited six months earlier, and his work was depending on his skills in equity lending. We had been like kids on Christmas morning with the gifts of his new opportunity, increased salary, and taking a step in the right direction with his career. Unfortunately, the events of September 11, 2001, started a morbid game of dominos that ultimately led Steve's new firm to lose substantial money, and Steve to lose his job.

The USA was shell shocked by 9/11, the financial industry tumbled and Steve felt the aftershock. On the world scale, his domino tumbling was very small, but to us, it caused significant damage. Despite receiving a generous severance package, Steve didn't handle the job loss very well and retreated from me emotionally. He left physically too. He regularly went out with the boys to cope with his perceived failure. We were already dealing with fertility issues and MS, now unemployment was added to the mix. Dr. Gaze explained to me that a man losing his job is akin to them losing his manhood. I was empathetic, but having just been diagnosed with a degenerative neurological disease I reasoned that Steve's job was replaceable, my health was not.

The sheer horror of what happened in New York that day coincided with me going through uncertainty with my health and I, like many others, couldn't seem to cork the tears while watching the TV. How could those people get on their elevator that morning and not come back down at the end of the day? Many years have passed and when I'm feeling low, or am complaining about this or that, I still think, "Yes, times are hard, but we're here. We have life, and a good life."

There are many things we can't control in life, but we *can* choose how we perceive things. Throughout my life, perspective has helped ground me.

—ɯ—

After my MS diagnosis, I didn't go back to the fertility doctor. Steve and I had to determine how my new disease was going to affect our lives and, more pointedly, my ability as a mother. During the first few months of learning about the disease, the thought of children became a question mark. By this time, I had two neurologists, Dr. Smith, and then, after my diagnosis, Dr. O'Connor. I had pushed my family doctor to get me in to see him because he was close to my home and ran a first-rate MS clinic at St. Michael's Hospital in downtown Toronto. I respected and liked Dr. Smith, but he was located in Mississauga, a suburb of Toronto, and was a general neurologist, not an MS specialist.

The two doctors had very different answers when I asked them, now that I had MS, would I be able to raise a child? Dr. Smith, always the more cautious of the two, said, "All the sleepless nights could be detrimental to your health."

I didn't necessarily trust his wary approach because I knew people with MS had babies. I appreciated his caution, but didn't want to give way to too much pessimism. When I asked Dr. O'Connor for his opinion about whether motherhood and MS could intertwine, he responded, "Of course you can still be a mother." I decided I needed to do more of my own research and come to my own conclusion.

I tried to figure out what my life was going to become. Would Steve want to be with me if I ended up disabled? Was I going to end up alone, with MS, and the dear auntie to my sister's children? I knew how much an aunt could mean in your life, so the thought didn't terrify me, but it did make me melancholy. The one thing in my entire life that I have been sure of is my love of children and that I would enjoy, and shine at being a mum. I have said assuredly on many occasions that motherhood would be my calling.

I had never been certain of my career path, and had subsequently fallen into jobs. My employment has been steady and I have always been a well-valued employee, but I've yet to find a job that says anything about who I really am. At one company, I was asked whether I wanted to take their management training program—apparently, they thought I was a natural leader. I said, "No, thank you. I don't want to have to fire anyone." I had no desire to be a boss. I was happy occupying less prestigious roles. Some of that was related to feeling uncomfortable being in charge. No Big Boss role for me. Motherhood, and the creativity and energy that make a good mum, were what I strived for. I had a great role model. My mum loved motherhood.

I wasn't sure I had the stamina for a demanding job and motherhood. I watched people do both well, but I had my health to consider. A friend helped Steve find another good job in his field at one of the big five Canadian banks and his salary gave me flexibility with my job choices; I was fortunate and didn't need to be motivated by money or ambition. I could stay home, or work part-time if I became a mum. Lots of men and women with MS have families and I was not ready to give up my dream of having our own family because I was saddled with this new neurological disease. Steve and I kept trying to have a baby.

Chapter 26

New normal

—∽∿∽—

"Hope is being able to see there is light despite all of the darkness."
—Desmond Tutu

In the first year after diagnosis, I was hyper-aware that I had MS. It was the dictator in my brain, ruling my thoughts. I was sensitive to every ache in my body. I became in tune with my legs. Were they sore? Were they fit? Were they twitching? Were they flexible? Were they deteriorating? Were they improving? The all-encompassing worry was exhausting.

Slowly, somewhere along the way, the twitches, the pain, the good days, became normal. I learned that every time my legs ached did not mean that a wheelchair was imminent. I figured out that my hormones affected my MS symptoms, so tracking my menstrual cycle became more than just about having a baby. I learned that I could still dance until the wee hours, and I would be only marginally more tired than pre-MS days. I learned that MS didn't have to control my life, but I needed to listen to the signals that my body would send to determine my limits. Numbness, tired eyes, toes that stuck together, stiff fingers, a tingly upper lip . . . all these things reminded me to put down one or two of the balls I was juggling, take a deep breath and recalibrate. I chose what I could and couldn't manage. I was editing out things that required too much energy for too little added value to my life. Everyone has to make choices for one reason or another; this didn't make me unique.

I continued to improve at yoga and, the next summer, I did 40-minute swims at the cottage whenever I had the chance. I practiced yoga on the deck in the early morning sunshine. I swam before the boats were out, and was back to the dock to see the first water skiers hit the lake. We had adopted a two-year-old Boxer dog, Dexter, and I walked with him daily. He was a kind, gentle, loyal, 80-pound companion. Most importantly, I enjoyed my exercise routine much more than when I used to be a gym rat. It was less of an effort now to become motivated; there was a very definite purpose to my exercise that wasn't just about having an attractive physique. I wanted a physique in good working order.

Throughout my life I have enjoyed being active. When I was a kid, it was gymnastics, tennis, skiing, horseback riding, and family walks. In my teens and twenties, I got into the eighties aerobics craze; and in the nineties, I spent a lot of time at the gym on the treadmill, Stairmaster and various other machines. At that time, I wanted to be strong, but my time at the gym was more about how I looked. My "fat-free" diet phase had only lasted for a couple of years, so I was slim, not skinny, when I was diagnosed with MS.

I had been puzzled after my surgery in the late '90s that I could no longer manage the Stairmaster, but now it made sense. So did a lot of other unidentified physical symptoms I had experienced over the years. For about 14 months when I was a teenager, I suffered from shin splints that couldn't be explained. I was told to ice them and reduce the jumping around I did in aerobics. That put a damper on my routine, but I adjusted my exercise plan. Then the pains mysteriously went away. Several years later, when I was on summer break from university I awoke and could barely walk because I had a searing pain in my hips. My hips were X-rayed to check for arthritis. The results were negative. I was prescribed an anti-inflammatory drug and told to quit the gym for a bit. My hips got better and life went on. I believe that these were two MS relapses that totally remitted. Research suggests that many MS patients have likely had the disease longer than they think. More and more young people are being diagnosed with the disease. Is this because of environmental factors, improved diagnostic tools, or that doctors are more aware of the disease? Maybe it's all of these things and more.

I recognized that my central nervous system would become agitated from extra stress, so I did a lot of yoga and spent most of my free time with my friends, or Court and her fiancé Brian. They were my cushions from the harshness of reality. My sister accompanied me to yoga and we enjoyed the spiritual and physical nature of the practice. It calmed me, strengthened my muscles, improved my balance, and was 90 minutes of time where I could empty my mind and get in touch with my body. We also found humour in the practice because some of the more complicated poses were making us into hilarious bendy straws. Even "corpse or resting pose" at the end of the class provided some comic relief. Courtenay would take her Zen to the level of snoring, and I'd have to give her a firm poke to wake her up.

Along with yoga, I decided to eat a gluten-free (GF) diet to try to reduce the inflammation in my brain. From what I had read, it would be good for my gut too. At the time, GF goods were not readily available at the major supermarkets so I was hauling myself all over town to get some decent pasta and bread. I was also taking some vitamin D and fish oil supplements to help combat the effects of MS. My neurologist had done a much-referenced research study on the benefits of vitamin D and strongly suggested taking daily megadoses of D, and didn't discourage me from trying other things. He said there was no scientific data relating to the GF diet, but he had several other patients who swore by it, and it couldn't hurt to give it a try. I agreed, and if nothing else, it gave me some hope and a perceived sense of taking a sliver of control over the disease. I was trying to be sensible about my expectations and was making life changes that I thought might help my symptoms. I was finding ways to substantiate my hope. Controlled hope is a powerful thing.

I was very encouraged that, after three months of adhering to my GF diet, the numbness in my feet disappeared. I also had more energy. This lifted my spirits and made it much easier to stick to my diet. I still had bouts of fatigue, and, if I was exhausted, my toes would stick together, but it was a lot less often. Also, the more I researched,

I realized that the perception of MS had been changing for several years. In the past, people thought MS would inevitably lead to being confined to a wheelchair. This isn't true. It can lead to immobility, but for over thirty years, there have been vast sums of money channelled into research, resulting in incredible breakthroughs in treatment options for people living with the disease. Many people, with or without the medications, live full and mobile lives. Some have very few symptoms, while others have to constantly manage their disease and their mobility, or lack of it.

For many patients, even though they "look great," they may be experiencing various invisible symptoms. This presents challenges. It can lead to fear that others think you are "faking it." I haven't run into this, but I know some people who have. One very common symptom of MS is overwhelming fatigue. Sometimes when the fatigue is at its worst, I look my best. I look fresh on the outside because I have to rest so much. It can make it hard to ask for help because it doesn't look like it's needed to the outside world. To keep a feeling of independence and potency I rarely ask for help. This has been a downfall of mine but, as I get older, I'm finding it easier to say what I need.

During this time, my relationship with Steve started to feel more fractured. Surprisingly, the months of our marital discord were free of MS symptoms. My hand felt normal and my legs strong. Steve seemed happy to be employed again. My job at a finance company was very busy, my days productive and my mind occupied. But I didn't feel like our marriage was a partnership. I spent a lot of nights without my spouse and managed my time and loneliness by seeing friends and family.

Chapter 27

Alone

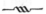

"If you want to keep a secret, you must also hide it from yourself."
—George Orwell

Aloneness was a familiar feeling for me. Over the years I had spoken with Dr. Gaze about how isolated I sometimes felt by my ileostomy and childhood experiences with colitis. I was all shiny and bright on the outside, but had experienced horrifying darkness and physical pain, so my inside was a jumble. I felt like an unread book with a misleading cover.

With Dr. Gaze, I was figuring myself out and learning to use my voice. I wasn't sure that most people really knew me, and if they did, maybe they wouldn't like me. I felt more complicated than my appearance and actions suggested, and indeed things were complicated.

From an early age, I decided to hide my ileostomy. As a family, we even hid my illness and surgeries from my grandparents in England and Scotland. My parents feared that my Grandpa Ireland would feel some sort of guilt about my genetics due to his Crohn's disease, and resulting colostomy. They thought this would be especially difficult for him because he wouldn't be able to tell me what he was thinking. My mum's mum had never liked my dad so we thought she would blame Dad's genes on my misfortune. Also, all four grandparents lived in the United Kingdom and would feel helpless.

Before my parents had decided to keep my health trials from my grandparents, I had written a letter to Grandma in Scotland. She was the one I was closest too, although, her husband, Mum's dad, was my favourite grandparent. The letter was never posted. Several years ago,

I found it unopened at Mum's house. I ripped it up without reading it. I still haven't figured out why I did that. I thought, "It's all over now, so I didn't want to revisit that chapter of my story."

I wish my parents had told my grandparents about my autoimmune disease and resulting surgeries because keeping the secret from them made me feel more distant from them; I didn't really feel that they knew me anymore. When I was around Grandma Ireland in Los Angeles, when Aunt Jill was sick, I saw her look surprised when my stomach made noises that must have been familiar to her because of Grandpa's colostomy. I don't think she guessed though. My maternal grandmother was a different story. She was very nosy. I am 99.9% sure that, while cleaning up at our house, she decided to tidy my (very neat) walk-in closet and found my ostomy supplies. She became strangely keen to tickle and feel my stomach. It was weird and I knew why. We still didn't tell her. I began thinking that maybe we should, but squashed the idea and just hoped she wouldn't confront me. I began to think that by protecting my grandparents, I had lost a bit of myself. I didn't dwell on it, not even years later in therapy. My parents did what they thought was right at the time, and I still understand why. I would do it differently today, and so would they. Hindsight. 20/20. You know how it goes.

During my school years, I lived in fear that my bag would make a loud, totally uncontrollable, fart noise during class, or that it would fill up at inopportune times. I remember once, in Grade 6, being in the library and our class was sitting on the floor while the librarian addressed us. Just as she was trying to get us all to be quiet, I could feel my stoma moving and was terrified that it would be noisy as it worked. Right on cue, as everyone obeyed her "Sssshhhhhh," my stomach made a long, slow, loud fart noise. I could have died. I know I turned red, but I just looked around at everyone else and tried to giggle with them as I feigned disgust too. Luckily, any smell was trapped within the bag, so even with all the bloodhound-like sniffing, the rude sound could not be traced to me. I emptied my bag several times a day so I was very self-conscious about leaving the public bathroom smelly on a regular basis. I know most people try not to poop in school bathrooms if they can help it. I had no option.

Hardly anyone knew about my bag and I was scared that people would think I was rude, stinky or less feminine. My bag was invisible underneath my clothes, but some of its "side effects" left me worried that my cover would be blown, or leave people bewildered by my sounds and smells. This caused me great anxiety then, and still does to some degree.

Dr. Gaze and I talked about my fears of being defined by my ostomy, and also of my shame. I told her about an experience with an ostomy support group soon after I first returned home from hospital. The hospital had presented the idea of meeting up with other kids who had ostomies. I would be the youngest in the group, but it still might be helpful to listen to how other people coped, so I thought it might be a good thing to try. Mum drove me to the meeting and waited in the hall as I went into the assigned room. Everyone was a teenager; that unnerved me, but didn't put me off enough to leave. I sat down inconspicuously at the back of the room and listened.

Sometimes our minds are selective in their memories and this is true for me about the support group session. I remember only one person from that meeting. He was about sixteen, lanky, with dark, greasy, stringy hair, and complained that his friends now called him Stinky. Everything he said was negative, but he lost me at Stinky. My brain shut down. I sat silently until break time, and then I went into the hall and asked Mum to take me home. I decided that I didn't need to be part of any support groups. I concluded that the guy clearly needed to take a shower and his ostomy probably wasn't why he smelled. I did not want to be part of a club that included him. It tapped into my biggest fear of being perceived as dirty. I determined I would figure things out on my own, with the support of my family and few close friends.

After all those years of keeping my bag under wraps, I decided not to hide the fact that I had MS. I sent an email to my boss moments after my diagnosis explaining why I had to leave the office for the day. My instinct was to reveal my new disease. I had lived with an invisible illness for my entire adolescence and adult life. With MS, I wanted to feel less alone with the fear, even if I wasn't talking out loud about the scary part of the disease with most people. At least they would know I was going through something.

My gut told me to be forthcoming about my MS and a big part of it was that I was tired of hiding something that had impacted me in such a major way. I didn't brandish a big "I have MS" banner, but I didn't make any extra effort to conceal my new disease. I knew how alienating that could be. I had been hiding my ileostomy for twenty years. What I realized later, after being so open, is that some people feel uncomfortable being presented with "ugly" information like disease, even if it's not related to going to the bathroom. By sharing the fact that I have MS, I run the risk that people will only see that, and I'll end up more invisible. I was, and am, willing to take that risk because the rewards are bigger than the pit falls.

I know I'm the farthest thing from alone, but sometimes, when I've been in a room full of people, I've felt as if I'm taking in the sights and sounds through a sheet of glass and am engulfed by the white noise of pointless conversation and forced laughter. It can be lonely to be surrounded by so many people, and feel so little connection to any of them. I don't even want out of my glass casing; I just want out of the situation. Sometimes I feel like nobody I love really gets it. I mean really gets it. And why should they? They're not in my body feeling the sensations that I feel. They're not in my mind filled with wheelchairs and intestinal turmoil. They take for granted that they can run across the street without having a leg spasm. They don't shit into a plastic bag on their stomach.

My protective layer grows when I am feeling tired or a bit defeated. I've learned to retreat from the social scene when I need to. Sometimes it's for a day, sometimes a week or two, but I always shed my Mylar coating and come back. If I don't take that time, I become trapped in my own numbness, surrounded by a white icy sheet of aloneness. I have so much support yet still am occasionally unsure of using it. I felt safest discussing my darkest fears with Dr. Gaze because I knew I wouldn't burden her or be judged.

I remember when the Tom Hanks movie, *Cast Away* was released in 2000. Steve and I went to see it in the theatre. Tom Hanks' character, Chuck, is marooned on a desert island in the South Pacific after he is involved in a plane crash. Chuck spends four years finding ways to survive, and copes emotionally by talking to a volleyball that was in the plane's cargo. He names the volleyball after its brand name, Wilson. Wilson becomes Chuck's avid listener, confidante and friend. Talking to Wilson keeps Chuck sane and hopeful. Wilson is always there. When Wilson is swept away by a wave, and gets lost at sea just before Chuck is rescued. Chuck is devastated, and I cried and cried watching the scene. Steve didn't understand why.

Chuck lost his best friend and a very good therapist, an avid listener. He was forced to figure out his own thoughts. In the end, Chuck is rescued and the last scene of the movie shows him at his Welcome Home party. He looks very uncomfortable and shies away from the crowd. He looks lost. People are greeting him like he is the old Chuck. I blubbered big, salty tears watching this. I knew that Chuck would never again be the same guy his friends had known. I got myself together to leave the theatre and then cried during the car ride home too. In my mind, Chuck was no longer on the island; he was the island. I identified with that feeling. Steve was dumbfounded as to why I was so upset. When I explained my grief, he was no less perplexed.

It was a catch-22; I didn't want to feel alone, but I didn't like voicing my true thoughts for fear of being judged as a downer or too needy. I also didn't want to dwell on things. I stayed positive by moving forward and keeping things in perspective by remembering the many good things in my life. I did my own Cognitive Behaviour Therapy long before it was a known coping strategy.

Not long after my MS diagnosis, my mum's friend Rita was diagnosed with breast cancer. They removed the lump, found lymph node involvement and suggested chemotherapy and radiation. This bright, vivacious, single 60-year-old woman stated that she did not want to have chemo. With no children or close family, she felt that there was no need to put herself through the gruelling treatments for only a possible cure. When my mum told me this my throat burned, but I couldn't cry. I wept when I was told Rita's tumour was cancerous, but couldn't manage tears for her aloneness. It was too close to my heart. The feelings were so familiar, but I didn't admit that I knew what she meant. I have a family that would miss me terribly if I died, but the isolation of illness is a powerful force and even your best friends and family can't completely lift you out of it. Maybe because I was struck with sickness so young, I always felt I had no choice but to fight. Choosing to let the disease win wasn't an option for me, but Rita had a choice and her first instinct was not to go to battle. Now that I'm a woman and no longer a child, I understand her choices and think that I would still always choose to wage the war for life, but I know how difficult the battle can be.

With all my talk of loneliness, it's an interesting fact that some of my most happy peaceful times have been alone or with animals. There's a lot written about animal therapy these days. I understand why. Whenever I am told to go to my happy place during a medical test, or for relaxation purposes, I think of horseback riding.

One of my best experiences horseback riding was in 1997, before my surgery to remove my stump. After Aunt Jill died, Uncle Charlie still welcomed our family to use the Vermont guesthouse and riding stables. When he wasn't there, he would ask his staff to make sure we had access to everything we needed. Being at the farm made me feel connected to my uncle, cousins and aunt, and being on her horses in the Vermont woods brought back wonderful memories.

During this visit I went for a morning horseback ride. The day was summer perfection: the air was hot, the sky blue, and the sun shining. A slight warm breeze rustled the leaves on the trees—the quintessential day for a trail ride. It was so perfect that it didn't feel real. I took great deep breaths to enjoy the smells of nature and the barn. After saddling up my favourite mount, Zurich, we headed to the galloping track, an expansive grassy field surrounded by the woods. The trails brought back memories of riding with Su and Aunt Jill and the pure joy she experienced navigating them at a full tilt boogie gallop, ducking when the horse took you too close to a drooping branch, and holding on tight when you jumped over a fallen log. I have always had the sense that the horses enjoy the woods as much as we do; it had to be a lot more invigorating than doing figure eights in the sand arena.

This day, Zurich and I walked the short distance to the track and I quickly realized we were not alone. Forty yards ahead, unaware of our presence, was a mother and baby deer grazing peacefully. Halting Zurich, I held my breath trying to make the scene last, and it did, for a dream-like minute. When the doe spotted us she surveyed the scene before leading her fawn back to the trees, disappearing into the cloak of green. How could I be so lucky to get an up-close look at Bambi and his mother, and share their world of the woods? For the second time in my life, I imagined myself in a Walt Disney classic.

Intoxicated by our sighting and charged with a new energy, we crossed and circled the field with a life-affirming vigour. We swerved, I ducked, Zurich kicked up his hind legs in gleeful bucks. He was full of piss and vinegar and I was too. I felt free; I felt enveloped in the deer's innocence; I felt part of nature. Feeling full of the magic of summer, I almost expected to float up to the clouds and ride around surveying the world below. That's how I imagined my spirit world version of heaven. When I close my eyes and remember that morning, even in the midst of winter, I can feel the warmth of that day and my chest feels full and my body light.

That feeling is like a drug. Forget Botox; charging through the woods on horseback is all I need to feel plumped with youthfulness and energy. When I ride, I feel light, but grounded and strong. I am part of the earth and the horse's energy comes right through the saddle and into my body. My body becomes part of its rhythm. There's nothing else that gives me this sensation; I can revisit it easily because it's so distinct.

My face and body glistened with sweat after a charged ride, my legs felt weak when I dismounted and I felt a quiet, all-encompassing bliss. With that pleasure was the knowledge that I was lucky. For all the horrendous experiences, there had been a plenitude of occasions when I had seen the opposite end of the spectrum, and I relished the times that had lifted me to heights of wonder and abandon.

It didn't get any better until the post-ride grooming. My helmet came off and my sticky head steamed in the air. My hair smelled like horse, and a layer of equine dust stuck to my exposed sweat. Perspiration trickled down my face, and I smeared dirt along my forehead and nuzzled the neck of the horse that was mine for that moment.

My nose had become accustomed to the stable smells, but after a workout in the fields we had both become more pungent. I wanted to wipe the smell of his coat on my body and breathe in the warm air that came from his nose when he sighed. The meaty skin of his muzzle was soft, supple and the big teeth hidden beneath did not frighten me. In the steamy moments after a ride, when I was shiny and the horse was glistening, time moved in slow motion. Protesting the flies, the horse beat his back foot like he was counting the minutes until the pesky insects disappeared. To dry off we walked around the barn, and I offered him some carrots in thanks. I had the pleasure of seeing a summer morning from his back and he had been an integral part of one of my purest highs.

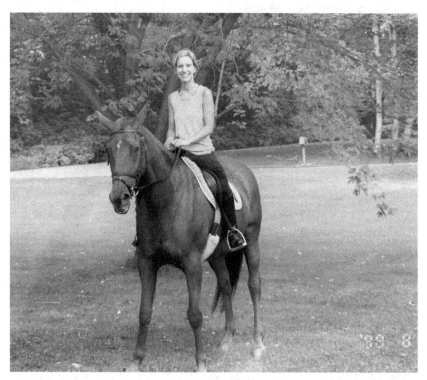

Me riding Zurich in Vermont. August, 1998.

Chapter 28

Eye am sinking

—ɯɯ—

"When you come to the end of your rope, tie a knot and hang on." —
Franklin D. Roosevelt

I am usually a "glass half full" kind of gal. Sometimes this positivity doesn't come easily. That's one of the aspects of MS that can be most distressing. I work really hard to stay healthy, and usually I win, with medications, supplements, discipline and a bunch of luck thrown in. This allows me to feel like I have some sort of control over the disease. But, during treatment for my first relapse, my glass was knocked over and spilt until it was almost empty, everything just a puddle on the floor.

It was the early spring about 18 months after my diagnosis when I experienced my first relapse, a bout of optic neuritis. I knew this was common for MS patients. I seemed to be looking through frosted glass in my right eye. I booked an appointment with my neurologist and he gave me the option of taking the steroid prednisone to "speed up the relapse recovery rate." I could also just let the eye recover by itself, but there was no telling how long that might take. Prednisone is a potent anti-inflammatory drug that should make the recovery process faster, but with no guarantees. I wanted to feel better for my sister's wedding in a few months, so I decided to take the drug. I was given a lot of prednisone intravenously as a child to try and control the colitis, but I hadn't taken anything remotely like it since. I associated it with having bloated chipmunk cheeks, but not much else.

Well, times had changed. I don't know whether it was because of all the bad memories still swimming in my head from when I was a teen, or if puberty had made a difference, but prednisone and I did not get along at all. Depressed is an understatement; I felt black. The lack of emotional clarity was disconcerting. It was like watching myself get lost down a long dark tunnel.

I attended a wedding shower for my sister during this time. I put on a good show for the event, but underneath I was struggling. Court's friend, Alison, was at the party too. A few months earlier she had been given a clean bill of health after battling non-Hodgkin's lymphoma. I knew Ali fairly well because her family vacationed in the same spot in Florida as we did. We had shared many good times on Sanibel Island. She's a lovely, pretty, kind, fun girl with a sunny personality. When I heard about her cancer, I sent her a note with one of my crystal necklaces that Aunt Jill had given me.

I saw her at the party and after giving her a big hug, asked her how she was doing. Ali still radiated warmth, but, like a soda pop that has sat out for a few hours, her bubbles were a little less fizzy. She inquired about how life was going with MS. I could tell she really wanted to know and I felt safe being honest with her. She had been to war too.

"It's okay, but I am on prednisone right now and am having a hard time with the side effects."

She took my hand and said "Oh, Lins, prednisone is the worst."

We said "I hate it" in unison and laughed.

As we shared our experiences we became absorbed in our own world; survivors, on an island for two. Ali knew the sensation of sinking into the abyss caused by prednisone. She had experienced the feeling of disappearing, getting sucked into quicksand and slowing sinking into the warm gooey muck. "You know it's the drug, right?" she asked.

I confirmed that I did, but she knew exactly how hard it was to remind yourself that you will come out the other side of this treatment as the person you recognize as you. We spoke the same language; it was eerie how similar our steroid sensations were.

The next day, during a crying episode, my mum tried to console me by reminding me that I bring my family so much joy. That seemed like the farthest thing from the truth, and I just cried harder. I was convinced that I was the family black cloud, and imagined what life would be like for the others with me gone. I fantasized that it would be hard for them at first, but then the relief of not having my health problems to deal with would set in and their life would be so much easier and brighter. It would take a while, but then the sun would shine, and their grief and their biggest burden would be gone—whoosh—into thin air.

I really had to fight these thoughts and push them from the front of my mind. When did this hopelessness set in? For the first time in all the years of seeing my therapist, she asked me if I was having thoughts of harming myself. I answered her straightforwardly. "It's not that I am having visions of doing myself in, but I am thinking that if I got hit by a bus, or struck by lightning, it would be because it was meant to be."

I felt as if I was dying anyway, so it would just be some sort of natural progression of the despair. If someone could just shake the hell out of me, and readjust my MS-riddled brain, I knew that I could get back to being me. I could again be the girl who brings, as my mum suggested, my family happiness—I knew the enthusiastic sister, daughter, wife and friend was in there and that the attack on my eye and prednisone was stifling my spirit and hope. But how could this feeling be temporary? It was overwhelming.

As I was nearing the end of the first prednisone treatment, my eye got better, and my mood improved slightly. I felt strong enough to utilize some of my usual tactics to take care of myself. I drank a lot of water to try and clear my system of any leftover prednisone toxins, upped my acupuncture appointments, saw Dr. Gaze weekly, continued with yoga, my GF diet, and used visualization techniques to meditate.

Chapter 29

No wish for death

"... I am a thousand winds that blow, I am diamond's glint on snow..."
—Uncle Charlie's grave stone

The fear really hits you. That's what you feel first. And then it's the anger and frustration. Part of the problem is how little we understand about the ultimate betrayal of the body when it rebels against itself." Uncle Charlie said these words about my aunt's cancer during an interview. I imagine he must have felt a similar terror as his mind gave way to dementia in the final years of his life.

In 2002, Su had given birth and wanted to spend some time at the farm with her dad to ensure that he met his new grandchild. My cousin's pregnancy had kept her from Court's recent wedding, so she asked us to come for a visit while she was in Vermont with her baby. I was looking forward to seeing Su and meeting her newborn, and I also knew it might be the last time we saw Uncle Charlie. Court and I drove nine hours from Toronto to the farm. Kim had renamed the property and made a few unfortunate changes to the main house, but most things remained the same.

When I entered the house, Uncle Charlie was sitting comfortably in his favourite brown leather chair with his feet resting on the matching footstool. For as long as I could remember, standing guard beside that chair was a four-foot tall, hand carved, Indian chief statue. He looked a bit like my uncle, but his sombre expression seemed almost sorrowful now.

Uncle Charlie knew who I was as he hugged me hello. He was quiet and looked grief-stricken as I talked to his wife, Kim, and their secretary, Sue, about the status of my MS. I had written him a newsy letter a few months prior telling him some details about my life and health; I'm not sure if he forgot about it, or if he ever got to read it. I held his hand, and looked him in the eye as I reassured him that I was doing well. I told him how happy I was to see him, and be in Vermont with Su and Courtenay, and that I was savouring the countless memories of family times together. His bruised hands clasped mine as he attempted a weak smile, but his moist, cloudy eyes looked pained. He had a hard time finding his words and called Su "Jill" several times.

Every inch of the place held memories for me, many of them with Uncle Charlie. He was always so physically strong, and, like the cliché, often silent. He knew a lot about nature and would enlighten Su and me by pointing out interesting things during lengthy walks in the woods. He was protective and would continually check to make sure that we were safe as we navigated the forest. One summer, when I was about thirteen years old, there was a man who worked at the farm who gave me a bad feeling. Most of the staff were long-time employees, but this guy seemed transient, like he wasn't interested in being part of the team. I don't recall his name or exactly what he looked like—he was kind of thin, pasty white and greasy but I do remember the uneasy way he made me feel. He seemed to skulk around and pop up when we didn't expect him.

That summer, Su and I decided to sleep in the "boys' room." It was on the opposite side of the house from her room and her parents' bedroom. My male cousins weren't coming to Vermont until very late in the summer, so we had their large bedroom to ourselves, with five single beds to choose from. As young girls, we had snuck into this room during many summer afternoons, when the boys were out, to snoop or short-sheet their beds. On Christmas mornings, suited up in their onesie pajamas, Su and Court had stormed this bedroom urging the boys to "get up, get up, get up!" The adolescent matriarch, I followed behind in my nightie, but was just as eager to get Christmas going. The boys, more interested in sleep than presents, greeted us with farts and fooled us with morning breath "secrets" blown in our faces. The room that had historically been off limits was now ours for the month. We each picked beds that were next to one of the large windows overlooking the front yard and horse pastures.

One night, I awoke at two in the morning because I could hear someone walking around the front of the house. I shook Su awake and we looked out all the windows to try and see who or what was causing the noise. It sounded like footsteps to me, but we saw nothing. Was the weird guy hiding out there? Or someone else? I felt like a fox being chased by the hounds; my body was lit up with adrenaline and my heart was pumping wildly. I needed to do something to ease my anxiety.

Aunt Jill and Uncle Charlie's bedroom was off limits to us unless we were invited in. They protected their privacy and sleep time, so I was afraid to wake them. On top of that, Su and I were scared to run from one end of the house to the other to get to their bedroom, but the terror of an intruder outweighed these concerns. I didn't stifle my fears, I was petrified.

With moonlight illuminating our way, we scurried across the house, and knocked loudly on their bedroom door. Uncle Charlie answered in his bath robe and listened as we rapidly outlined our concern. He disappeared to put on some clothes. Moments later, he appeared in a grey sweat suit, Nike sneakers, toting a handgun. Aunt Jill clutched the sheets over her naked bosom as she sat up and said "Be careful, Charlie." I had never seen a gun up close before and, until then, I didn't know Uncle Charlie kept one in his bedroom—that added a level of excitement!

He walked us back to our room and then went outside to patrol the perimeter of the house. We watched what we could from our bedroom windows. My uncle was measured and deliberate in his search for what, or who, might be out there. He didn't find anyone or anything near the house that shouldn't have been there, but he didn't make me feel silly for being scared. Vermont was Uncle Charlie's safe and happy place, he wanted it to be ours too. The worker who seemed shifty didn't stay on the farm until the end of the summer. I never knew whether he quit or was fired.

I have a deep love and appreciation for nature and some of that was taught to me by Uncle Charlie, in Vermont. He wouldn't have understood walking through the woods with headphones on; the sounds of nature filled him with peace. He built Su a tree house from scratch on the top of the hill at the edge of the woods, that overlooked the back of the main house. He took immense pleasure in picking blackberries for his morning granola cereal. I would watch his strong hands sort through the fruit to discard any that were past their prime. He rarely seemed rushed, in contrast to my dad who got up early and picked up a buttered bagel on his way to work each morning.

Lately, I have wondered what Dad would have been like if he had ended up the successful actor in his family? He loves nature and animals, especially horses, as does my mum. As a kid, every Sunday Dad and I would watch the popular nature television show *Mutual of Omaha's Wild Kingdom,* an educational series based on the lives of animals. Dad knows a tremendous amount about a wide variety of creatures. If he had had vast resources of time and money, I can't picture him on motorcycles like my uncle, but I can imagine him riding horses as a pastime. Being a successful actor allowed Uncle Charlie many months of family time, away from a working schedule. His life was so different from my dad's and other men I knew, but I didn't reflect on that at the time. It was the Bronsons' normal existence and, by extension, my summer standard.

When we were with Uncle Charlie, we didn't wait in line at Disneyland or at restaurants, and strangers would wave across the street at him, sometimes calling his name. Some would give him a thumbs up. It seemed as if they knew him, but their familiarity was based on his celebrity, nothing else. He was modest, so liked to stay home a lot and preferred the quiet of Vermont to the bustle of Los Angeles. I was just a kid and didn't really understand how popular his movies were until later. I was into romantic comedies and musicals, not vigilantism and cowboy flicks. I still haven't seen many of his movies. When I was in university, several of my guy friends had posters of my uncle on their dorm room walls. That took me by surprise! I was completely taken aback when I visited the local video store to rent a movie and saw two life size cut outs of Uncle Charlie displayed near a section of action films. I could have high-fived his cardboard hand, although the semi-automatic weapon he was holding would have made the exchange clumsy.

It was a revelation—he was a hero to my friends, and to the male public in general. I never said a word about my connection to him, except to a few of my close friends, and they didn't make a fuss. It's not that I wasn't proud of my uncle, I was. I kept silent because of loyalty to him and my cousin, Su. She had recently changed her name, and since elementary school, had been suspicious of some of her friends' intentions. She worried that they mostly liked her for her Hollywood status. I had no desire to cash in on that allure. It would have felt like a family betrayal.

Uncle Charlie was eighty-one when he died on August 30, 2003. He knew where he wanted to be buried and had bought a big plot at the Brownsville cemetery in West Windsor, Vermont. His gravesite is at the top of the grassy hill that overlooks Mount Ascutney ski hill. We spent many days as a family on those slopes. The ski resort closed in 2010, but, luckily, mountains stand proudly with or without people swooshing down their inclines. Only a couple of close business associates and family were invited to Uncle Charlie's funeral. Dad, Mum, Court and I drove to Vermont to be with our cousins and Uncle Charlie's wife, Kim. The sun shone brightly as his mahogany casket was lowered in the ground. I was blinded by the sun and my tears throughout the short service.

Kim arranged a family dinner after the service, and my cousins and I ended up singing songs from our childhood and reminiscing about many good times with my aunt and uncle. Uncle Charlie's death felt like the end of an era. It was mildly surreal at the time and my memories of it are hazy now. I said goodbye to Uncle Charlie that trip, and also to the Vermont house, pond, woods, trails and horses. Katrina, Su, Court and I had one final day lounging by the pond, and I swam laps around the island. My uncle had been the one to holler at me when I swam crooked on my back, and ended up in the middle of the pond. This time, as I self-corrected my path, I laughed at the memory. Like she knew what my younger self would have loved to hear, Katrina said "Lins, your body looks phenomenal! Su, doesn't she look great?" So many years around that pond, with so many body issues. I don't think she had any idea of the emotional dynamite that was packed into her comment. I wondered if the spirit of my aunt or uncle put those words in her head.

A year or so later, when Steve and I adopted our Boxer dog, Dexter, I asked myself if my attraction to, and affection for, pug faced dogs was related to the quiet loyal love of my Uncle Charlie. Many movie reviews described his pug-faced looks and the fact that he was ruggedly "ugly-handsome." I thought of my uncle as good looking and I have a visceral reaction to all squishy faced dogs that is hard to explain. I love their looks. They feel like family. I want them in my family. Dexter was quiet, calm and communicated so much through his eyes. I loved his strong body and the way he joyfully bounded through wooded trails and grassy areas. I took comfort in the way that his looks intimidated people. He was a total pussy cat, but looked like a bad ass. It seemed very familiar to me and made me feel safe.

Chapter 30

It's a boy!

—ᄴ—

"Encourage and support your kids because children are apt to live up to what you believe in them." —Lady Bird Johnson

It's a boy. I immediately melted at the news, and felt like my insides were gooey, warm, yummy chocolate. It was a delicious feeling. I don't know why, but I had been expecting a girl. Girls were all I knew; my sister and I were what would be considered traditionally "girly." We played with dolls, loved crafts, clothes, shoes, interior decorating, and our Easy-Bake Oven. I barely made a cake in that toy stove, but used it as a testing centre to melt many non-food items. I loved exploring, animals and being outdoors and active, but shied away from team sports, and much to Steve's disappointment, I didn't even watch sports. I was going to be a mother to a boy. I was elated!

In April 2005, about five years after we started trying to become parents, our son was born. Holding him in my arms, looking into his perfect little pink face, I was in rapturous awe. Later, he bawled his eyes out while the nurse gave him his first bath. I was scared he would get a chill because, judging by his protests, he was freezing. My anxieties quelled when he was clean, swaddled, calm and snoozing. Aaron was the most beautiful baby I had ever seen. I was completely smitten.

It was a bright, chilly day when we left the hospital the next morning. Steve and I handled Aaron like a rare Faberge egg while loading him into his car seat. I had a ton of babysitting experience, but nothing quite prepares you for going home with an infant. Aaron slept for several hours at a time and awoke for feedings. He was easy except that, like a lot of babies, he had his night and day mixed up. Most of his alert time was in the very early hours of the morning. Dr. Smith's warnings of fatigue were on my mind, but I knew I would rest when I could.

I took Aaron for long walks in the day and made sure he was well bundled. It didn't matter what time it was, I sang "Mr. Moon, Mr. Moon, you're out too soon, the sun is still in the sky" to an enraptured Aaron. When the song was done, if I wanted to keep him awake, I'd babble away asking him rhetorical questions or explaining what our two cats, or Dexter were thinking. "Dexy is wondering when we'll go for a walk, he loves to chase squirrels and see his doggie friends in the park." Yes, I was becoming one of those women. I didn't want to chase (evil!) rodents, but I did want to get out for our walks and chat with people in the park. As wonderful as motherhood is, it can be a bit isolating.

If it was time to sleep, I'd rock Aaron in my arms or in his portable swing. I worked on trying to keep him awake for longer periods during the daytime so we could establish a sleep schedule in the coming months. Come 7 pm, I'd announce, "It's story time" and Aaron and I would cuddle in bed as I flipped through picture books, with him sometimes trying to grasp the pages. He became accustomed to stories at bedtime, and it was an important part of our routine. During the day, we would sit on my bed together while he lay on his play mat, or while we looked at the pages of his hardcover books, him sucking on the corners if I got distracted. Later, when he learned to sit up, the books became another source of entertainment. Yanking them all of the shelves into a heap on the floor became a great source of fun! Fun for Aaron, reloading the bookcase became a tedious task for me. I nicknamed Dexter, Shadow, because he followed our every move closely. With Aaron strapped to my chest in the Baby Bjorn, the three of us would take in the sights while I did my errands.

I wanted Aaron to grow up feeling secure, loved, and with a healthy self-esteem. I was set on exposing him to as much as I could so he could choose what interested him. It was important to me that Aaron felt protected, but as he grew, he would also feel enabled to try new things to expand his horizons and feel safe, even if he failed. Like most mothers, I thought Aaron was the smartest, loveliest, most

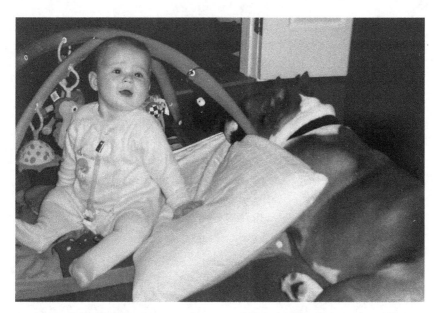

Aaron on his play mat with Dexter laying close by. 2005.

beautiful baby I had ever seen and I aimed to be a relaxed mum, but with a healthy mix of intentional parenting.

Four months earlier, Courtenay had given birth to the first of my parents' grandchildren, Liam, so we were thrilled to be new parents together, and the boys had built-in playmates. We had our matching Boxer dogs, identical strollers and baby boys. We bought them coordinating pajama sets and took tons of photos of our newborns. Court and I saw a lot of each other during our maternity leaves and enjoyed watching our boys grow, discover their worlds, and each other.

Both of our sons took very well to sleep schedules, so I had lots of time in the day to rest, keep house, put together photo albums and correspond with friends. I had few MS symptoms and enjoyed long walks every day with Aaron and Dexter. Between women stopping to admire Aaron, and men stopping to say hello to the dog, my walks weren't always speedy, but they were social.

As the weather warmed up, Mum and I went up to the cottage with Aaron and Dexter, and Steve joined us on the weekend. I would nap with Aaron in our screened in porch listening to the birch trees rustle in the breeze. When dinner time came, and Aaron got fussy after his feeding, Mum would meander around the small garden, holding him in her arms, telling him about all her plants. Her banter and the sights and sounds always calmed him. I was a poor audience for her flower talk, so she appreciated Aaron's rapt attention. I walked the hilly road daily, pushing Aaron in his stroller, swam when he napped and kept up with my yoga. I'd never been more fit.

After my maternity leave, Steve didn't want me to go back to work. He grew up in a very traditional household where his mother took care of the four children, did the cooking and kept the house clean, while his dad worked and controlled the finances. My upbringing was slightly different. My mum had done the accounting for the family company as well as looking after the family finances. She was a good cook, but didn't get to utilize her skills very often because Dad was basically obsessive-compulsive in his cleanliness and tidiness. He didn't like the house smelling of food, or the mess that meal preparation caused, so we ate out almost every night. My other experiences with family meals were in Vermont, a cook made the meals and the kids ate in a different room than the adults, so at least when it was the four of us, we were all at the same table, even if Mum and Dad usually talked about his business.

As Dad's business grew, we had a weekly cleaning lady, Dad still helped with the laundry, and Mum continued to take care of the garden. I was aware that Mum suffered from empty nest syndrome when Courtenay and I went to university, so I aimed to avoid that and keep one foot in the work force. To maintain a work-life balance, and not become overwhelmingly tired, I found a part-time job after Aaron was born. It was a 5-minute drive from our house, accommodated my need for mental stimuli outside the home, brought home a paycheque, and satisfied my desire to be a hands-on mother without becoming exhausted and sick.

Chapter 31

Salon therapy

—∿∿—

"Exchangeable, interchangeable, substitutable, switchable..."
—Synonyms for *replaceable*, Merriam-Webster dictionary

As any woman with a long-time hairdresser knows, your stylist can fulfill the need of therapist from time to time. My hairdresser, Pete, has seen me through some pretty vulnerable moments in my life. He has diabetes, so we both understand the world of autoimmune diseases. He regularly asked me questions about my MS, what I do for exercise and how I manage my symptoms. I always spoke openly about all these things and nagged him about his diet and to quit smoking. It took me years to tell him about my ileostomy. It was just another example of me keeping it under wraps, even from the guy who saw me with a head full of tin foil.

I had shared some of my marital frustrations with Pete at various past appointments. Now it was 2009 and my marriage with Steve was ending. We had become parents four years earlier, but Steve had not become the family man that I had hoped. Unfortunately, he seemed even more restless after becoming a father. As a new mother, I could no longer avoid the fact that Steve was often unreliable or absent, Aaron was my first priority. The problems in our marriage magnified because I didn't just have me to think about anymore. As I faced our marital issues head on, I had to make a heart-breaking decision.

As I was deciding to end my marriage, Pete got a lesson on the despair of divorce. Four little words was all it took; "How are ya, Lins?" he asked as I sat in the swivel chair to begin my hair appointment. His question was so mundane. The answer is usually automatic, polite and predictable. But that day my eyes welled up, and my mouth began to quiver as I bit down on the fleshy part of my upper lip until it disappeared behind my teeth in a vain effort to stop the slow leak of tears. It was not a dramatic howling—there were no histrionics, gulping, or waterfalls—just a slow measured drip of sadness. I had cried all the way home from yoga the previous Saturday. My sunglasses shielded my eyes, but nothing could hide the salt-stained cheeks. Everyone gets the blues sometimes, right? Maybe for a couple of hours, a day...or two, but this had been four solid days of me feeling like I might blubber at any given moment. Not since my episode with prednisone had I felt like this. Something had to give and the safety of Pete and his salon chair enabled me to let it out and then collect myself.

Instead of reading a gossip magazine I took the time under the heat lamps to think back on how one of our final marriage counselling appointments had been pivotal.

—⚊—

I was deeply unhappy in our marriage. I was talking to Dr. Gaze about how I felt, but that only addressed my feelings, not Steve's worrisome behaviors. "I feel unheard. He's just saying what he thinks I want to hear but doesn't show any signs of changing. Last night he said that I'd never leave because of the money." I shook my head in disbelief. "He doesn't know me at all."

Dr. Gaze responded in her usual calm manner. "How do you feel about that?"

I felt a melancholy that was rooted in the pit of my stomach. I said, "I think counseling is our only hope. I can't do this on my own."

She countered, "yes, but how do you feel?"

I didn't want to sob; I knew we only had a few minutes left. I choked out, "heartbroken, my chest actually feels heavy and achy." I started to quietly weep and reached for a kleenex to wipe away my tears.

A few days later, I asked a trusted friend for the name of a marriage counselor. Later, I confronted Steve. "It isn't negotiable," I said. "We need to go if we have any hope at saving our marriage."

He immediately bristled; "Oh, great, I bet you have found someone who will take your side and the two of you will gang up on me."

Did he think I was a playground bully or this was some sort of game? I explained that I hadn't even spoken to the therapist; no plotting had taken place. If this felt like a sport to him, he wasn't used to losing. An excellent athlete, his trophies had always meant a lot to him.

At the time, my husband's firm was involved in a complex lawsuit and Steve was being coached on how to respond to corporate lawyers—he spent hours training and it was paying off, just not for me. He was getting slicker during our arguments. He said less, revealed little, and always remained calm. Our discussions became circular and would lead nowhere; it was infuriating. He was clearly paying attention to his coaches and adapting legal strategies to our home life. My husband had already revealed that he felt he had the upper hand due to his earning power, I wasn't sure of much that would make an impact, but as I said to Dr. Gaze, I needed to know I tried everything. I didn't get married to get divorced.

We decided to drive downtown together for the first appointment with our therapist, Cathy. Steve arrived home from work, didn't have time to change and as usual, politely opened the car door for me as we prepared to depart. The radio played two Katy Perry songs in a row, "I Kissed a Girl" followed by "Hot N Cold." I wondered out loud if the singer was in town for a concert.

Steve replied, "Why are we doing this? You know I don't want to do this."

We were at a stoplight and I looked out the window onto the street. I felt trapped in the car. The sidewalk was teeming with people. Happy people; sad people; people who were excited to get home to their families and some who weren't. Continuing to gaze at the street, I replied, "We need help if we are going to find our way; if we are going to stay together. We need to be able to talk to each other. Hopefully, Cathy can help us with that."

Cathy's practice was in an office building. By 7 pm the building was quiet, as was the waiting room. Steve and I sat beside each other on the couch; he picked up a magazine, I didn't. I scanned the room and took in the dark hardwood floors, Oriental rug, the Monet print on the wall, and the tall leafy plant in the corner. I started wondering if Aaron had eaten all of his dinner. My mum was babysitting so I knew they would be having a good time. I had nothing to worry about at home. By now, the tub was likely full of bath toys with Aaron creating streaks of "fishies" with his bath paints. What was Steve thinking about? His poker face didn't give anything away, although his tapping right foot belied his nerves.

The office door opened revealing a short, attractive blonde lady wearing a navy-colored suit that I thought I had seen at Banana Republic. She looked more business-like than Dr. Gaze, but seemed very pleasant and welcoming. "Hi there, I'm Cathy, come on in." We introduced ourselves and each settled into a wing back chair covered in a dark velour-like fabric. They were comfortable. That was important because our first appointment was 90 minutes, double the time I spent with Dr. Gaze, but there were two of us talking, so the extra time was understandable. Steve and I faced each other, with his back to the door and mine to the big window. Cathy's chair was, fittingly, in between, our mediator.

I knew this appointment would involve getting our family histories and explaining what we were hoping to achieve with therapy. I wasn't nervous; I was chomping at the bit to get going. I was desperate to see if someone could help me crack Steve's shell. I'm not sure what I thought we'd find, but I was desperate for some forward momentum.

When Cathy asked us to describe our childhoods, I learned that being the youngest of four children, Steve had sometimes felt neglected. His mother had four children in four years so I imagine she was exhausted. He remembered long hours in a playpen while his mom watched soap operas. I knew his mom to be very industrious, but if anyone deserved to have suffered from some post-partum blues or fatigue it would be her. That was a lot of youngsters to care for, by herself. Steve's dad was busy at work all day, running his cable company. Cathy was a good listener, and Steve a better patient than I had imagined.

I was practiced about talking about my past, so shared what I thought was important. My time at SickKids definitely factored in but I spoke about my family too. When Cathy asked what brought us to see her, I explained that I felt I was in the marriage alone. I received a lot of apologies from Steve about late nights, over indulging and forgotten phone calls, but nothing changed; I was losing respect for my husband as well as self-respect by allowing myself to be treated so carelessly. She took notes and asked how Steve felt about that.

"I'm here because Lindsay wants us to be here." His honest reply was disheartening, but Cathy seemed charmed. On the drive home Steve told me "That wasn't so bad, I just told her what she wanted to hear."

Our homework was to go on a date. We went out to dinner at a neighbourhood Italian restaurant, and I kept thinking Steve would prefer to be out with his buddies at a bar. Was he just here because we had booked a second session with Cathy?

Steve seemed more confident on appointment number two; he knew what to expect. He had a bit of his usual swagger and Cathy seemed almost star struck. Was she flirting with my husband? Surely not. I must have imagined the coquettish look in her eyes.

However things moved along at this appointment I found myself confessing, "I think Steve may be subconsciously mad at me. My final ostomy surgery had complications that lasted months, I was diagnosed with MS five years after we were married and I had fertility issues. I'm a bag of broken toys. Maybe that's why he stays out so much and needs to drink."

Cathy looked at Steve and asked, "Do you have anything to say to that." He looked me square in the eye, and very calmly stated, "I am just an asshole, and it has nothing to do with you." Cathy gave me a look that said, "See?" Steve continued, "You are the nicest person I know, you're hot, you are a great wife and mom, I never cared about your ostomy or your MS. I am just an asshole."

I was quiet. He was telling me what I suspected, but that didn't make it easier. I genuinely wondered, "What am I supposed to do what that?" Steve shrugged. I don't remember the rest of the session because I was reeling. Nothing else was said that has stayed with me. Shockingly, we made an appointment for the following week. I needed the counseling time to try and extricate myself from the marriage with as little collateral damage as possible. I started to quietly get myself prepared to leave.

At one of our final appointments with Cathy, she warned me, "It's hard out there in the singles world." She seemed to be working for Steve. In my head I was thinking "Maybe for you. Marriage is no joy either." Out loud, I said, "I know" and did my best not to look at her like she was crazy. I wondered if in a few months' time I'd hear that she and Steve were dating.

I snapped out of my reverie when Pete announced "Time's up, Lins. Let's get you washed and conditioned."

"Sounds good, Pete. Looking forward to being blonde and root-free again" I chirped. I was feeling stronger than when I had entered the salon, but the fact remained that after being with Steve for sixteen years, thirteen of them married, I was going to be on my own. This was the cause of all my earlier grief; but that's not all. I was the one who had to end it. That prospect was daunting. I had some control of this situation and the pain that was going to be inflicted on Aaron, Steve and me. I was not used to that.

Hurt had not eluded me in this life, but generally, in the past, I had no influence over the situations. I had no control over the surgeries, the death of Aunt Jill, my parents' divorce, and the MS diagnosis. All I could do was figure out the best way to manage through the calamities that struck. Some coping strategies were innate and intuitive, and some very calculated. Therapy, change in diet, exercise, support systems, so many things to choose from. I did have control over what happened in my marriage, and it was time to make a change.

That word really resonated with me. Control. What if, with all this control, I messed everything up, and ruined the rest of my life? What if my instincts were wrong? What if I ended up lonelier and more alone than I already felt? And poor, too. What if Aaron ended up hating me? There were so many things to be scared of. But, when I allowed myself to think of the reasons why I was preparing to leave the safety net of my marriage, my intuition told me I was doing the right thing, for me and for Aaron. I had to believe, and trust that, with time, my world would be brighter, I'd feel lighter and maybe even have the energy to extend myself in ways that I previously had not.

Even after all our marriage counselling and very forthright conversations, Steve didn't really think that I would leave. He was very upset to be wrong and wasn't used to losing. I think that's what it felt like for him. He didn't just lose me and us, he lost the image that our life portrayed. We had an adorable, sweet, healthy child, a nice house in a family neighbourhood, a cottage on a lake, an SUV, the mountaineer stroller and handsome family dog. The list goes on, but I think I'm painting a familiar picture. It all seemed very white picket fence–ish.

Steve's parents were distressed by our separation. His mother called me in tears. She asked if there was any possibility that I could find a way to stay. I explained what had taken me a while to figure out; I had lost respect for myself and because of that I was losing my integrity. I couldn't live a life where I had to spend so much of my time pretending that I was okay with our relationship. She seemed to understand. Over the years she had told me the many compromises she had made as a wife and mother, most of them very common in the 1950s, and I'm sure she only shared half of them with me. After our divorce, the few times that I saw my ex-mother-in-law she was nothing but kind and interested in how I was doing.

You might think feeling undervalued would be an obvious reason to leave my marriage. It wasn't. I thought a lot about staying and reworking my life in an effort to be happy. It was what I had done for several years. Before being a mother, on the weekends, I met my girlfriends for yoga and/or brunch, and by the time Steve got up, I had already enjoyed a healthy, social interaction. I had good friends, as well as my family who filled my need for meaningful and reciprocal support. I had stopped searching for it in my marriage because I filled the void elsewhere. I was patching the holes in our relationship with scotch tape. It wasn't enough to hold it together.

I was terrified of leaving our marriage. I was almost forty, had MS, an ileostomy and was mother to a four-year-old son. I figured it would take someone very unique to want to hitch themselves to my broken wagon. I thought I might never find them and I wasn't in the headspace to look for them. I was very busy and my brain was on overload figuring out how I would manage my new life on my own. I wasn't sure how I would handle some of my needs but, once I decided to leave, I made sure that I had a good support network for Aaron and myself.

I started filling my toolbox. Steve was the main bread winner and Aaron and I were on his benefits plan. My MS drugs were very expensive and, at the time, I worked for a small, not-for-profit organization. After explaining my situation, my boss told me to research benefit plans for small businesses so that we might find a plan that would work for our unique situation—two full-time and two part-time employees. I had tremendous support from every angle of my life.

I was very worried about Aaron's comfort, emotionally and physically. Where would we live? My dad, mum, sister and friend Jen, all invited me and Aaron to live with them. It made the most sense to live at Mum's house. She had the room, wanted the company, and it would be the least disruptive to anyone.

I knew we could never overstay our welcome there. She didn't think of charging us rent, but I wanted to contribute, so I bought the groceries and cooked. We moved in during the spring of 2009 and stayed until June 2011. Mum is exceptionally flexible about having people in her space. She likes animals too. We had Dexter and a leopard gecko in tow. Unlike me, or my father, some extra clutter and mess doesn't faze Mum. She would have liked us to stay indefinitely, but that wasn't in the cards.

I'd never been on my own before. I'd had serial long-term boyfriends since I was sixteen. Then, I married one of them at twenty-six. Now, thirteen years later, a few months before my fortieth birthday, I had decided to leave the comfortable institution of marriage. Institution isn't a warm, nurturing and cuddly concept. Hospitals are referred to as institutions too, and I knew well the pain that can live within the confines of those establishments.

Interestingly, once I was on my own, many women asked me in confidence how I had managed, because they were unhappy in their marriages and were thinking of leaving. I absolutely did not want to be the Divorce Poster Girl. There is nothing fun about divorce. I made sure that people understood that, and unlike most single mothers, mine was a very cushy story. I had a lot of support, a lovely free place to live, and large child support and alimony payments that I could save for our future. Also, sometimes marriage counselling works. If it does, it could be worth the considerable effort. If that fails, it is important to make sure you are ready to be on your own. The best advice I could give to anyone thinking of divorce was to be prepared and realistic. I told them not to count on a white knight swooping in and saving the day. Life isn't a fairy tale.

I was devastated and terrified when I decided to leave my husband. People said "things will get better," "this too shall pass," "time heals all wounds," etc., etc. . . . . That's all true, but as I rode the emotional roller coaster of splitting up, whenever I felt stronger, I reminded myself to store some of my buoyancy for whatever challenges lay ahead.

It was about three months after my separation from Steve that I learned he had met someone new. I felt heartbroken. I had left him, and was well ensconced at Mum's house, and supported by the rest of my family and friends. Why did I feel overcome by grief? I couldn't understand my tears and the hollow feeling in the pit of my stomach. I cried gut-wrenching sobs in the bathtub. The tub and me—why is it my favourite cry zone? Water begets waterworks?

At my next appointment with Dr. Gaze, I explored my feelings. I knew divorce was devastating, but it wasn't just about that, I was having a hard time articulating what had triggered all this sadness. I had thought I was all cried out. Dr. Gaze had me examine my fears about Steve's new girlfriend. She had two kids, a girl, slightly older than Aaron and a boy four years his senior. I was worried Aaron might prefer being with Steve's new tribe, and leave me behind. Furthermore, even though I didn't want to be married anymore, it was difficult being so quickly and easily replaced. I wasn't angry, and intellectually I knew that men usually don't like being alone, but I was melancholy and that feeling had taken me by surprise. Dr. Gaze pointed out it would be rare for someone to immediately feel happy that their former spouse had moved on. Being replaceable is not easy to accept. As I shared my fears of Aaron "trading up" to a family with siblings, Dr. Gaze listened and then asked me about my own experiences. Never once would I have exchanged families. She assured me that from what she knew, Aaron was well mothered, and that a safe and secure mother-child bond is not easily replaceable. It didn't take me long to feel happy for Steve that he had someone in his life. The bathtub went back to being a place to bathe, and not a place for a sudsy sob.

Chapter 32

e-Harmony

—∽—

"You are only afraid if you are not in harmony with yourself." —Herman Hesse

Somewhere near the end of my first year living at Mum's, people kept asking me "So, are you dating yet?" It's like after you get married, when everyone wants to know when you are having kids; they just assume it's the next step. I was open to the idea of dating, but wasn't sure where I would meet anyone. I was living with my mother, didn't go to bars, worked from home, drove my son to school and his activities, walked my dog several times a day, and would socialize with my married girlfriends. I wasn't "out there." I was healing and rebuilding from a stressful couple of years, and enjoying my new routine. My dad repeatedly suggested that I'd meet someone in the grocery store. How would that would happen? I couldn't picture myself hanging out with the zucchinis trying to look alluring.

A good friend suggested online dating. She explained that there were a couple of sites that were geared towards relationships. I listened, and looked at a few websites. It took some convincing because I was nervous about putting myself online.

So, after a few nudges, I joined the dating website e-Harmony. I filled out their lengthy online questionnaire with brutal honesty. I didn't want to waste time going on dates with people who were unsuitable for me.

I had a few dates here and there, and saw one guy a few times. A couple of men were very keen to move forward, but, for various reasons, they didn't appeal to me. I had a match that I ignored for a while before responding to it. When I did finally reply, I moved at a turtle's pace, and we emailed back and forth a bit before I agreed to go on a date. Through our emails, I learned that, when he was a teenager and young adult, his parents had owned a house in Vermont, he had grown up near me in Toronto, and he seemed family-oriented. He had tragically lost his older brother in his teens and his adopted sister had been missing from their family for years. I reasoned that this man had experienced heartache and would hopefully have some emotional depth. I needed that quality. I was consciously trying to break past relationship patterns. My match, Chris, was eager to connect in person and, after several weeks of emails back and forth, I was too. We decided to meet for a drink at The Rebel House, the local favourite pub near my mum's house.

It was May 30, and we were experiencing a warm spring so I wore my favourite white halter-top, tight knee-length jean skirt and Mexican beaded sandals for our first date. Chris picked me up at Mum's house, and I was putting the garbage to the curb as he approached the house. I had seen him park his sports car sedan, and liked the look of him. He showed up in a golf shirt and shorts and had a tan that suggested he had spent some time on the links. In my flats he was at least five inches taller than I and his short, black, coarse, hair didn't add any illusion inches. He seemed relaxed when he introduced himself and had an easy smile. I liked his brown eyes. Aaron has brown eyes, so does my dad, and so did my dog, Dexter. We walked around the corner to the pub and were seated in the covered backyard patio at a table for two.

We had a lot in common and had many mutual acquaintances. I don't think this happens very often when using a dating website. Chris played squash and, through my university friends, I knew many of the guys on his squash circuit.

After our first drink, Chris asked me if I had time for dinner. Things were going well, and Mum was babysitting so I said yes. Chris excused himself to go the bathroom. Later I found out that he was cancelling another drink date he had scheduled later that evening. While I was dipping my toe in the dating scene, Chris was seriously looking for a serious girlfriend.

I liked Chris's approach to the date. Socially, we were at ease with each other, but he didn't want to waste his time, or mine, if our life-styles and goals weren't compatible. He fired off a lot of questions. At times it felt like a bit of a job interview, but I respected that he wanted to know if we were on the same page about real-life things.

Chris's two daughters were in their teens so he first asked, "Do you want more kids?"

Go big or go home. I responded easily, "No I'm one and done. I feel very lucky to have Aaron. No more babies."

I'm pretty sure I saw his shoulders relax at my response. At thir-teen and fifteen years old, his girls were well passed the baby stage. From my perspective they might make good babysitters. I laughingly said, "Judging by your body language, you aren't looking for more bambinos."

He responded, "I can't even imagine going back to the diaper stage."

Aaron was well out of diapers, but I thought it was important to remind Chris, "Aaron just turned five so he takes up a lot of my time. He is my first priority."

Chris seemed to understand that and moved on to what felt like a random question, but I later figured out it was connected to my love of the cottage.

"So, Lindsay, do you enjoy camping?"

We were done with drink number two now, so I felt quite relaxed.

"Camping, like with a tent? No. Actually, hell no. I like a bathroom and a comfortable bed. If I'm using up my weekend or vacation time, it doesn't need to be the Ritz, but at least a form of glamping."

If he's a camper, this date was done.

Chris laughed as he replied "I hate camping." He then ordered another glass of wine. He liked camping even less than I did so we were good to go there.

Chris continued with his inquisition, "Do you prefer a hot or cold location for vacation?"

I laughed out loud and told him, he was a very earnest interviewer. I thought the question period was funnier than he did, but he was getting a kick out of it too. He was a high-level people manager at a bank so I guessed he was doing his "needs assessment analysis."

It was an easy question for me. "Sun and surf are best *pour moi*. I hate winter. I really feel the cold."

He smiled as he responded, "Me too, I despise it. I'm so glad you feel the same, I thought you might like ski holidays."

I let him know, "I did when I was younger. We skied as a family, but as an adult, I'd always choose a beach and I love the ocean." Check check. Beach man has found a mutual beach lover.

The talk about skiing led us to talking about our shared love of Vermont. Chris had spent time there as a teenager because his parents had owned a house there. I told him about how much the "Green Mountain State" meant to me because of all of my time spent there during my childhood summers and Christmases. I didn't mention that my aunt and uncle were famous even though I was pretty sure he'd know who Charles Bronson was. I had posted a picture of me riding on the e-Harmony website and Chris told me that he had been worried that I would be a "riding snob.". That thought hadn't occurred to me when I posted the snapshot. I just wanted to show people that I was active and liked animals.

As the date went on, any questions regarded smaller details.

"I see you like white wine." He noted.

"Yes, I love the taste of red, but it doesn't agree with me. I can't sleep if I drink it." I joked, "one glass or five, it doesn't matter."

He preferred red wine, but that clearly wasn't going to be a stopper issue. Several times throughout the date, I managed to work into the conversation that our kids were at different stages and that Aaron was very young and needed me. His dad was involved in his life, but I was the primary caregiver and I was very concerned with making sure that Aaron felt safe and secure. Chris seemed to understand where I was coming from.

When the cheque arrived, I offered to go halves, but he declined, and paid the bill. Later, Chris told me that I was the only woman he had taken for a coffee, drink, lunch or dinner who had offered to pay. I couldn't believe it, but apparently, I was an anomaly in the dating world for men. Chris' wallet had been sitting on the corner of our table throughout dinner. It was beyond battered. I told myself "Whoa, girl" as I thought about buying him a new one for Christmas.

After our dinner, I saw Chris driving away with a big smile on his face as he did a celebratory fist pump. This guy wore his heart on his sleeve; it was refreshing. It made me smile too. A few hours later, I was tucked into bed watching some mindless TV, when "ping," I received an email from Chris stating, "I had a great time. You've exceeded my expectations. Would you like to go to dinner?"

There would be no game playing here. I instinctively knew that he didn't mean to be funny, or managerial, but I giggled as I typed out my reply. I stated that I was clearly having a really good week—I had just received the same "exceeded" review at work. I accepted the dinner offer and we made a plan for date number two.

I was excited as I waited for Chris to pick me up. It was another beautiful pre-summer night, and I wore a cute, sleeveless black top with gold studs around the neckline and dark skinny high-rise jeans that made my legs look long. Green patent platform sandals completed the look. When Chris pulled up, he immediately told me that I looked nice and we drove to a restaurant that I occasionally used to frequent with my former colleague from Holt Renfrew. I told him this, and, as I explained that I had worked for the president, we realized that I had met Chris's dad, Iain. He had been on the Board of Directors at "Holt's." What a small world! I could feel our excitement bubble up as we eagerly chatted about what we both knew of my former boss, Holt's and my memories of Chris's dad. It was energizing to realize that we shared yet another connection. We already had a spring in our step, now we were practically hopping to the restaurant.

While getting ready for our second date, I had decided that it was important to tell Chris about my MS. If it was going to be a deterrent in moving forward then it was best to get it out of the way. For some reason, I didn't get stressed about explaining my MS to Chris. I waited until the main course and then just told him. I answered some basic questions about the disease and how it had affected me so far. I hadn't had any very severe relapses, but that didn't mean that I wouldn't in the future. I stressed the fact that MS is unpredictable, I didn't want to sugar-coat the disease. I also suggested he look it up online and then ask me anything he had questions about. Outwardly, it didn't alter the flow or feel of the evening in any way.

Our next date was a few days later at Chris's house. Aaron was with his dad for the weekend, so, on the Saturday evening, I went for a BBQ with Chris and his daughters, Caitlin and Stephanie. We had a good time playing Monopoly on his back deck and after a while the girls went upstairs to their rooms. I thought this was the right time to let Chris know about my ileostomy. I was forty years old and had never been rejected because of my bag, but I was deeply nervous about sharing this information. On our second date, Chris had told me that, years earlier, his mum had recovered from a bout of colon cancer so I silently wondered if she had had a temporary ileostomy; many people do when cancer is removed from their colon. If she had, then he might know a little about ostomies.

Looking back, I'm trying to remember why I split sharing my two health issues into two dates. I could have just spilled it all out at our second dinner. Did I worry it was too much for Chris, or me? My guess is that I needed to see his reaction to my MS, to build up enough trust to share the thing that made me feel the most vulnerable, my ileostomy.

In my younger years, I usually needed "liquid courage" to tell a potential suitor that I had a bag. I was stone cold sober when I took advantage of a break in our conversation to tell Chris I wanted to talk to him about something. I felt like my eleven-year-old self when I re-entered the classroom after my first surgery. I was insecure and wanted to blend into the background. I wished I could be sucked right into his comfy couch. I didn't know how to be me. I thought this might be the guy who wouldn't want me because I poop out my stomach into a plastic bag. I had been anticipating this rejection my entire life as an ileostomate.

I remembered one day when I was seventeen, I got home from school and there was mail for me on the kitchen counter. Mum was puttering about as I opened an envelope with no return address.

Inside was a card shaped like a cruise ship. It was an invitation to join a cruise full of single people with ostomies, and the tag line of the event was "Meet your Osto-Mate."

I started laughing uncontrollably. It was more like a maniacal cackle. Mum looked concerned. I think I may have seemed a bit deranged, definitely not like I was unleashing great joy. I handed her the card, and as I collected myself, I expressed some frustration and anger, but looking back on it, I think a lot of what I was experiencing was fear and hurt. Did people out there think that single people with ostomies would only be loved and accepted by other people with bags? I felt insulted. At the time, I had a lovely, kind, handsome, boyfriend who didn't give my ostomy a second thought, so I huffily tore up the invitation.

Guys are so visual. Didn't my aunt teach me that all those years ago when she bought me the sexy lingerie? Even though the evidence of my past experiences did not support that my bag was a turn-off, my mind went straight to that memory. What she, and more importantly I, failed to recognize is that the bag is only one small part of me. The rest of me is quite appealing visually and moreover, the bag is not so ugly either, it's just a bit of skin-coloured plastic. Still, I worried that even though in the past, my partners had found me sexually appealing, maybe this would be the one who wouldn't be able to see past my ostomy.

I was sweating profusely and my brain was having a difficult time arranging the words to tell Chris my big dark secret: the body that I had wrapped up in tight, attractive clothes had a big blemish and it was dead centre of me. Chris was compassionate and encouraged me to say what was on my mind. I can only imagine what he was speculating. I was looking left, right, up and down, anywhere to avoid making eye contact. I mopped my brow with a nearby napkin. Finally, I took a deep breath and blurted out that I had an ileostomy, and did he know what that was? I exhaled, and I think he did too.

To my great relief, he did know about ostomies, and I wasn't going to have to describe the details of what my bag did for me, which was the part I dreaded the most. I was right, his mother had lived with one for several months as she recovered from colon cancer. He took my hand, told me to calm down, and judging by his slightly confused look, clearly didn't understand why my revelation was so hard for me. I felt foolish, and also relieved that my secret was out in the open. My sweat dried and my heart rate returned to normal. I was emotionally wrung out, but recovered quickly and we enjoyed the rest of the night chatting, and shared some sweet kisses on the couch. We laughed as we caught Chris's eldest daughter, Caitlin, trying to spy on us from the kitchen, and I went home knowing that Chris now knew all my medical conditions.

The next morning, Chris texted me to see if we could meet for breakfast. I liked that idea, so we met at a local greasy spoon for eggs and bacon. As I tucked in to my Eggs Benedict, Chris apologized to me for not asking more questions about my bag and for seeming insensitive. I hadn't felt bothered by any aspect of his behaviour; I had been too worried about melting into his couch and disappearing into a puddle of shame. Chris also asked me why it had been so much harder to discuss my bag than my MS. It didn't make sense to him. MS is an unpredictable and potentially debilitating disease so, theoretically, it should give a potential long-term partner more pause for thought. Intellectually, I agreed with him, but emotionally I had not yet come to terms with the fact that people wouldn't reject me because of my bag. More importantly, if they did, I didn't know how I would handle it.

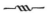

Years later, a friend told me about a national news clip that referenced a gorgeous girl who has a website called uncoverostomy.org. The woman's name is Jess Grossman and she posts pictures of herself online with her ostomy in full view. On her website, she's quoted to say, "I can do anything anyone with a full set of intestines can do!"

I was thunderstruck by these images and the whole idea of widely sharing one's ostomy. Jess replicates famous model poses or ad campaigns, with a bit, or a lot, of her ostomy showing. I did more googling and discovered she's not the only young lovely person out there displaying their ostomies to the world. There were many young men and women proudly showing off their ostomies. There was not an old man in sight.

Uncoverostomy.org "is an online awareness campaign working to break the stigma surrounding ostomy surgery." When I first read that, I was blown away. I don't surf the Internet much, so I was unaware that images of It Girl Ostomates were just a click away. The exposure to this was overwhelming. I didn't know how to describe the associated tidal wave of feelings. I felt like I'd had the wind knocked out of me. I kept thinking that my experience would have been so different if this had been around when I was young.

I was sixteen years old one summer in Malibu when I floated the idea to my aunt Jill of exposing my bag to the outside world. I was thinking of buying a bikini and letting "my bag hang out." I had fantasies of strolling down the beach in a bikini with my ostomy in full view. There was a part of me that didn't feel obliged to cover it up and wanted people to see all of me.

Aunt Jill kindly advised against it. She was going through chemo and was almost bald. She rarely wore a wig and I admired and respected her exposing her baldness. Everyone knew she had cancer and still thought she looked beautiful, including me. I think my aunt's advice to forgo the bikini and "bag baring" was sound. Everybody knows about cancer and understands it. I'm not sure that the Malibu beach surfers and California teenagers would have been the best test audience for my coming out.

I wasn't seeing Dr. Gaze anymore when I first saw Jess Grossman's website, but I was so perplexed by the feelings that surfaced when I looked at the ostomy images that I imagined her asking me to describe how I felt about uncoverostomy.org. I couldn't. My thoughts and feelings were so jumbled. There was a logjam in my brain trapping my words. It was too much for me to dislodge and process; I'm still working it out.

Seeing gorgeous young women and men expose their ostomies with such confidence left me incredulous. The funny thing is, I have a body that society deems acceptable. I have always been complimented on my figure. The problem is, I didn't ever believe my body was beautiful—it had betrayed me medically so often. I want to love my body, but I'm not sure I'll ever be able to trust it enough for that.

As I've aged, I've been able to separate the mistrust of my health from the distrust I had of people's reaction to my body. It used to feel like I was pulling the pin in an emotional grenade when I told people about my bag. I would wait for an explosion of rejection. I don't have that anxiety anymore. I have told more people about my ostomy in the last couple of years than I have throughout the rest of my life. I have been pleasantly surprised by how many people know about or know someone with an ostomy.

I look at the ostomies in the online photos and can identify with the pain and suffering that the person went through to end up with a bag. I'm talking about physical and emotional anguish. I see the bag as a badge of honour and resilience. I don't associate it with beauty. It's linked to distress for me, and is difficult to view online. What do people see who don't have ostomies? The bag doesn't look gross in real life, so it doesn't look disgusting in the photos. Maybe people just think "huh, neat," or "That chick is hot, anyway," or even, "Cool girl," period. I think demystifying ostomies is brilliant, and showing them in sexy images is ground breaking, and when I was younger, I think it would have done some good to see the photos. Now, I feel sad that I spent so many years with the narrative in my head that would be titled coverostomy.org, and was filled with shame and fear, instead of pride and openness.

Chapter 33

Onwards

—◦◦◦—

"Just remember, once you are over the hill you begin to pick up speed."
—Charles M. Shultz

I was as fit as a fiddle when I met Chris. I was seeing a personal trainer once a week, doing yoga and living an active life. I felt strong and my body had some muscle definition. When my sister and I got together, I'd jokingly flex my biceps because she had given me the nickname "Pipes."

By doing weights at the gym, my strength was measurable, and I was encouraged that I had increased my muscle by hard work with my trainer, Dan. He made me feel confident by continually challenging me with new exercises. The gym assigned Dan to me, and he was a great fit for me because he understood my limits due to MS. But more importantly, he figured out how much I actually could push myself. Dan helped me overcome my fear of the machines at the gym.

It was also really important for me to learn to do the exercises correctly so I didn't do myself more harm than good. After several years of following an exercise routine that included walking, swimming and yoga, I wanted to make sure I was taught proper techniques for using the equipment at the gym. I was proud of myself for safely pushing my limits to see what I could achieve physically and was pleasantly surprised with what I accomplished. There were days when I overdid it and I suffered from intense fatigue, but I treated those as "learning lesson sessions," took a few rest days and then got back to work.

—᠊ᨺ᠊—

I had successfully navigated leaving my marriage and was feeling physically vigorous. I felt I was doing a good job at mothering Aaron through a precarious time. I was juggling a lot of emotional balls and did not feel overwhelmed. After a year of dealing with divorce lawyers, worry, and settling into a new normal as a single woman, I was leaving behind the fear, uncertainty and sadness that had weighed me down. I felt lighter and had more energy than before. It was easier to enjoy things in life. I loved taking Aaron to school and his various classes, I wanted to see my friends, and I enjoyed working part-time from home. I was exceptionally grateful for the life I was living, and knew that I was making decisions that were true to myself. Turning 40 had brought me new confidence. I felt womanlier, less girly. When Chris and I decided to become intimate, I was more comfortable being naked than ever before, and I became even more at ease as our relationship flourished.

Sometime after our third date, before we had been to bed together, Chris called me and told me he had something to share with me. This was after I had sputtered and stuttered out that I had an ostomy. He seemed very nervous over the phone, so I was ready for some big news. I braced myself. Is he missing a penis? Does he have another girlfriend? Is he still married? Is it worse than my ileostomy?

He was drawing it out, so I finally said "Just spit it out, it's ok."

A moment later I heard, "After you told me about your ostomy, I wanted to tell you something I am embarrassed about."

There was silence, so I figured he needed another prod "Ok, don't worry."

Then in all seriousness he said "I'm hairy."

What? I couldn't help myself, I laughed, and then apologized and said, "I noticed you had hairy legs, I've seen you in shorts and a t-shirt. It's no big deal. Are you kidding me, I shit through a bag on my stomach."

He replied, "No, my back is really hairy. I don't like taking my shirt off at the beach."

He was serious and I didn't want to be rude, so I tried to empathize as he continued.

"It has always caused me a lot of stress and messed with my confidence."

I don't think he was just trying to make me feel better about my bag. He was worried about me seeing his body naked.

I couldn't really understand his concern, but I said, "We all have our hang-ups for our own reasons. I've seen hairy men before and I'm not the least bit concerned about it. Thanks for sharing that with me though. I could tell it was hard for you."

He replied, "Thanks for being so understanding."

"No problem, really, it is not an issue for me."

Before we hung up, we made a plan for when we would next get together. Sharing our vulnerabilities so soon in our relationship helped connect us as a couple.

After dating for about a year, Chris and I were ready to take the next step, and decided to move in together. Several months before meeting Chris, I had set aside some money to buy a house for Aaron and myself. I hadn't seriously started looking, but had removed some money from the stock market to ensure that I had the down payment available when needed. I was on the lookout for potential properties as I drove around the city and would casually look at things online. I was getting ready to leave my mother's nest for the second time in my life.

After his divorce, Chris had stretched his budget and bought a detached three-bedroom house, turned a room in the basement into a fourth bedroom/apartment, and had a renter living in the basement to help pay the mortgage. After some discussions about finances, Chris and I decided that I would match the equity he had in his house and we would share the mortgage payments and bills. Chris gave his renter two months' notice, and we started preparing our children for the transition. We then had a lawyer draw up a document detailing that I owned half the house.

I'm very pragmatic and practical and didn't want to risk losing any of the money from my divorce. Life had shown me that things don't always work out as planned, and I do what I can to mitigate complications. I didn't want to leave Aaron and myself exposed financially. Chris and I were in agreement with how we should proceed and we moved ahead, drawing up wills in the process. Chris had no furniture in his living room and dining room, and I had wanted Steve's apartment to feel like home for Aaron, so had given most of my furniture to him in our divorce. Mum still worked part-time at a lovely furniture store, and the owner extended his staff discount to me.

I bought some living room and dining room furniture, and we also used some things that I had been keeping in storage. The new furniture was more contemporary than Chris's girls were used to, but they liked it when everything came together, and we mostly hung out in the TV room, which had their old furniture. I was dying to change the paint colour on the main floor, but held off so Caitlin and Stephanie didn't feel like a tornado had entered their lives and wreaked havoc on their space. It would take a long time until that house felt like "ours." I referred to it as Chris's house for well over two years. I would correct myself, especially in front of Aaron, but, because I didn't choose it, that home never quite felt like me.

Chris's teenage daughters came and went from the family home based on a schedule with his ex-wife, and Aaron did the same. Many of my friends rolled their eyes when I told them Chris had teenage daughters, implying that I was in for a wild ride. Once again, I felt fortunate in life; Caitlin and Stephanie did not display the histrionics that I hear about from other parents of teenagers. They were welcoming, although I'm sure the transition was hard for them in many ways. If it was a distressing time for them, they kept it to themselves and certainly did not take it out on me, Aaron or Chris. Things went smoothly, I was still working from home, and Chris's house was no further from Aaron's school than Mum's place, so the logistics were easy too.

It was important to Chris and me that we try and regularly make time for just the two of us as we forged ahead in building our new life together and blending our families. I think because Aaron was so young, it was more important to Chris than me, but only because I was very uncomfortable leaving Aaron. Luckily, my mum, dad and sister were always on hand to help out and Aaron was with Steve every other weekend and two nights a week. I tried to schedule things based on when Aaron was with his dad. I loved my time with my son and thought that consistency in his life was very important. I wanted him to be able to rely on my presence. To me, that meant leaving my cell phone on vibrate when we were at the park, reading together every night in bed, a regular bath time, and being home as much as I could when he was with me.

Chapter 34

Hard to part

—ᴍ—

"Grief is what tells you who you are alone."   —Gail Caldwell

When Chris and I began making our life together, things felt stable; emotionally and physically. Neither of us had planned to get married again, but after several months of living together, we both changed our mind. There was no big romantic proposal—I think we both confessed "I want to be married to you," during a conversation about how lucky we felt to have found one another. So, we talked about it a few times, told our families and set a date for a small, intimate wedding. We were excited, but in a low key, level-headed way.

I felt secure and strong enough that I decided that I no longer needed my appointments with Dr. Gaze. I didn't feel like a bunch of disconnected mismatched dots anymore. It had been gruelling work at times, but our appointments had begun to feel like a habit, or a luxury, instead of a mental health necessity. Ending our appointments wasn't an easy decision; she had been my doctor for a long time, and a big part of my life, but I was ready. Although our relationship was professional in nature, our connection was deep rooted; its core was based on honesty, intentional learning and kindness. Our pairing was so tied to my emotional growth that it didn't feel simple to give it up. Like many relationships, the end felt like I was saying goodbye to a part of myself.

I've always been terrible at goodbyes. I get teary at airports when I see other people saying their farewells. Parting scenes in movies bring on the waterworks. I sob uncontrollably for the loss of other people's loved ones. I still held my breath a bit when Aaron left every other Friday to spend the weekend with his dad. I didn't have bad nightmares anymore about my son not making it home to me, but it took years to get over these fears. At the time, I couldn't figure out why it was so hard to say goodbye to my psychiatrist.

Dr. Gaze believed in taking time to say goodbye. When I knew I was ready to end our therapy relationship, she insisted that we carve out seven months for me to complete the process. I wasn't entirely sure what that meant. She reassured me that I would know.

She was right. After 22 years together, she understood how I was put together. It was she who guided me through all the puzzling pieces that were me. It took some time, but I understood the connections as they clicked into place.

So, why was it so hard to say goodbye? Dr. Gaze had taught me to honour and process good and bad feelings; I didn't think I was scared of the goodbye, but maybe I was? I was getting antsy about it. Three sessions before our specified end date I was feeling the heat. I didn't want an extension, so I took a deep breath and plunged in.

We started our appointment with the usual hellos and then I got to the point. "So, I'm usually pretty good at figuring out my reactions to things. You've taught me well. I know I am supposed to be saying goodbye but I am finding it hard to do. I know I am ready to end therapy. Why is the goodbye so hard?"

Her response was not a surprise, "What are your thoughts?"

Right. I had to figure this out. She wouldn't just tell me. Even at the end that didn't change. Too bad, I would have liked an easy "gimme."

I didn't think I had any relevant thoughts, but I kept talking anyway. "I can think of what it's not. I don't think it has to do with my parents' divorce. I don't think it has to do with my Aunt Jill's death. I don't think it's about my divorce."

She didn't say anything so I continued, "I have explored and mourned those really big meaningful devastating goodbyes."

She nodded and asked "Anything else?"

I smiled as I said "You obviously have an idea and I have to get to it. I don't think it's about being sick. I mean, I didn't die. I recovered. We've talked about all of that so much and I've shed copious tears for the little girl who was me. It can't be that."

Dr. Gaze raised her eyebrows slightly as she said, "You can't think of anything?"

There was a long silent pause—those were not uncommon or particularly uncomfortable. I was stuck so asked her for some help, "Seriously, any hints?"

She threw me a line, "Do you have any thoughts around your surgeries?"

My surgeries.

Oh my god. I blinked. Stunned. I felt like I was looking into that bright light that hung over the cold operating table.

I knew.

My brow furrowed as I responded, "How could I have not seen this? It's being taken away. . . ."

I became engulfed in the memory and began to sob silently. A minute passed and it wasn't so silently anymore. I decided to try to keep talking and clutched the wet balled-up Kleenex like it was somehow giving me strength.

I continued, "It's when I was eleven years old being rolled away in my hospital bed for surgery. I'm not sure if I'm coming back." I was having a hard time talking through my sobs, so I stopped trying to talk and just cried.

I had been looking at my lap, but looked up at Dr. Gaze as I said, "There was nothing light about being in The Hospital for Sick Children's pre-op area when your child is at death's door. My mum looked really pale and thin."

I took a moment to stop talking, blew my nose and wiped my eyes before I continued, "It was truly horrific. Horrifically terrifying. Mum, Dad and Aunt Jill all had a hand on me like they didn't want to let go. It was the scariest goodbye of my life. For them too, I think, because I was very ill at that point." Thirty years later the memory still unleased grief in me. There was silence as we looked at each other.

Dr. Gaze's voice was soothing as she prodded, "Anything else?"

I replied with a wry smile, "It explains a lot about the goodbyes. But I don't think *you* are going to die." She smiled and I continued, "I guess what's weird about this relationship is that I have revealed all of myself to you, but I barely know anything about you and I may never see you again. It's very final."

There was a long pause. It was up to me to keep going; I said, "The difference is that, even though we are saying goodbye, everything you helped me with will continue to shape who I am. You helped me find myself. You have been a huge influence in my life—I should say, a great influence. We are a really good team. I was one of your first patients so I imagine we both grew together. Nothing of what we did will ever die for me, but the end of it feels so final, sort of like a death."

I saw the sincerity in her eyes when she told me, "I'll miss you too."

Up until that moment, I hadn't let myself think about that part, missing Dr. Gaze; losing the connection to her. I replied, "I kind of know that. You have made it clear along the way that you like me. Is it ok if I send you wedding photos?"

"I'd really like that." She smiled.

I realized that this was the start of our goodbye and took the opportunity to say "If I ever write that book I've been talking about, you would be one of the first people I'd want to read it. Same goes for the stuff you said you might write. I'd want to read it." It seemed I was figuring out ways to ensure we didn't completely disappear from each other's lives.

She smiled as she said "Absolutely."

We paused and I looked at my watch. I realized that there were only a few minutes left of our session.

I said "Looks like time is up."

Dr. Gaze asked, "Are you ok? We can continue this next week. Let me know if you think you need any extra time."

I knew I don't need any extra time. What I needed to do was take what I had learned over our years together and forge ahead with my life. I had a lot of things that I wanted to do, so moving forward was my plan. Saying goodbye to the weight of past traumas had been hard work, but had allowed me to slowly heal and to recognize who and what I am.

I felt emotionally equipped to deal with whatever came my way, good or bad.

Chapter 35

Antigua

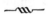

"Life is tough my darling, but so are you."   —*Stephanie Bennett Henry*

In February 2013, Chris and I booked six nights in Antigua for a romantic getaway. I was excited but, as always, anxious about leaving Aaron. I had been feeling a bit more tired than usual in January, but life had also been very busy, so I just pushed through.

Mum was in Florida for the winter, and Steve was unemployed at the time, so Aaron was staying with Steve while we were in Antigua. Although Aaron was well set up, whenever I travel without him, I am always irrationally apprehensive that the plane will go down and he will be left motherless. A lot of my anxiety was related to my illnesses and having to deal with so many complications with my health, especially as a youngster. Most kids feel invincible and take their health for granted; I didn't have that childhood luxury. Almost all my surgeries resulted in infections or complications, so I have come to expect, and plan for, a bumpy road.

The spot we had booked in Antigua was pretty. I felt very tired on our first full day, but put it down to travelling. The next day I woke up and my right hand was numb and weak, like it was before I was diagnosed with MS. This concerned me, but I wanted to be optimistic and focus on the sun, sea, Chris and me. I tried to think positive thoughts, but in the back of my brain I knew something wasn't right.

The next night, I awoke at two in the morning with a searing pain at the base of my neck. It was excruciating, and Tylenol and Advil did nothing to alleviate the suffering. I had never had pain associated with MS before, but I knew it was MS-related. I guessed that I had lesions in my spine and that something had activated them. I moaned as I writhed around the bed, and Chris tried, but could do nothing to help me. Just being there was all he could do. I was gripping and massaging my neck, trying to erase or squeeze the pain away. Then, for about 30 minutes I had trouble swallowing and began gasping for breath. I could feel my eyes bugging out of my head in terror. I had flashbacks of being confined to a hospital bed and my NG tube choking me. The visions were blindingly bright, razor sharp and scary and I couldn't duck the assault. It felt as if intense metallic bolts of lightning were scorching my brain.

I thought I might be dying. I was petrified. My mind raced with morbid thoughts. *What if this is it? Aaron! No. Find your breath, find your breath, don't choke, slow down, and remember to use your brain, find some calm and cling to it, you can breathe. You are breathing; slow it down, don't gasp. Keep your cool, take some air in, and then out. Any air is still a breath. Shut your eyes. Concentrate.*

I used my inner voice to find a way through those minutes and slowly my airway opened again. The relief was immeasurable, and it made the pain more bearable. I was thankful I could deep breathe through the searing bursts of agony to try and preserve some measure of calmness. A couple of hours later the pain abated and I passed out from exhaustion.

I awoke in our hotel room early the next morning, feeling shell shocked, and realized my right hand had lost all dexterity. It took me a minute to remember where we were.

My legs were heavy and clumsy as I found my way in the dim light to the bathroom. As I leaned against the counter for support, I tried to brush my teeth but couldn't hold my toothbrush properly. Combing my hair was awkward too. I knew I needed to contact my neurologist and get back to Toronto. I wanted to go home before it got any worse.

I hated being so far away from my family. It was a huge effort to walk to breakfast that morning; I had to concentrate really hard to make one foot go in front of the other. I wasn't limping yet, but it was a tremendous effort to walk properly. I couldn't write, or use my knife and fork. Although I couldn't use my hands and my legs were not working well, I looked normal, albeit a bit slow walking. My body had broken down overnight, but no one could see the damage. Again, the fear and suffering were invisible. I felt completely vulnerable as Chris cut my food for me. I think he was hoping I would spontaneously get better and we could stay but I knew that wasn't an option. This was the worst relapse I had ever experienced, by far. We emailed my neurologist and he confirmed that I could come to the MS clinic as soon as I was back, and he'd arrange for a nurse to give me prednisone intravenously at home.

We left Antigua the next morning. I needed a wheelchair at the airport. I could walk, but it took an extraordinary effort to do so, and my legs were very weak. I saw people giving me funny looks and figured that they thought I was playing the system to avoid the lines. I wanted to explain MS to them and tell them that the disease can take young, healthy-looking people and knock them to their knees. I knew people with canes, walkers and wheelchairs face pity, contempt and either too much or too little empathy, but now it really hit home. I had my own fears about being wheeled about that went back to being deathly ill, so my head was swirling with macabre thoughts of shame, sadness and anger.

I was worried about Aaron seeing me compromised, as well as the nurse coming and going from our home. My son was still so little. He was only seven years old and I didn't want him to worry about me. I needed to be his rock, not the other way around. Chris had a lot of flexibility at work so between him, my sister, Steve and my dad, Aaron had rides to and from school for the week that I was receiving prednisone.

I set myself up in the day on the main floor, and had the nurse come after Aaron had left for school. I only had to drag myself upstairs at bedtime. I rested and slept all day and then was able to have dinner with the family and get Aaron ready for bed. I wrapped up the IV port on my arm so it just looked like a boo-boo to Aaron. He told me, with a certain pride in his voice, "Mummy you look like a Transformer."

Chris and I had planned to go to Florida for March break, and despite my condition, I was determined to still get there. I needed to see my mum and be with my sister and her family. Building sandcastles and playing in the surf with his cousins would be a wonderful distraction for Aaron. I wanted this for him, and us. My legs were still weak and Chris was washing my hair, shaving my armpits and legs, and cutting my food because my right hand was taking its time to comply with the remitting part of the relapse. Emptying my bag took ages—this one-minute task could easily take me 15 minutes and be messy. One of my biggest fears for my future with MS is becoming dependent on someone else to take care of my bag. It hasn't ever come to that, yet.

After the Antigua trip, it took me over 10 days of rest and steroids before I could do five minutes of seated yoga arm exercises to try and make my hands meet each other over my head. They wobbled all over the place as I tried to control them. I felt like a marionette, with someone else pulling the strings. I did this every day until I could add another minute and then included some gentle seated leg movements.

I needed to finish my IV doses of prednisone before I could go anywhere. I would be able to travel once I started the pills that weaned me off the big intravenous doses. Courtenay and Brian offered to fly Aaron down to Florida with their family and look after him at their rental house for the few days before I could travel. Mum would be around to assist them when needed.

Chris and I changed our flights and left a few days after Aaron. I made the responsible decision to request a wheelchair at the airport because my legs could not manage the March break line-ups. Even if I managed to stay upright in the lines, my leg muscles would be completely depleted. I put aside my pride and did what made sense. I wanted to save whatever strength I could muster for Aaron, Chris and my family. Also, I needed to conserve my energy to do the work of finding potency and balance in my body again.

In Florida, I continued with my daily seated yoga sessions on the living room floor of Mum's condo, adding a movement every few days. After a week in Florida, I managed a short walk on the beach. Being in a sunny climate with my family was restorative; I was moving in slow motion but my tiny steady improvements made me hopeful. I rested a lot, but the days were filled with laughter and Aaron was so busy with his cousins that he didn't realize how much I was napping. A week later, when I got back to Toronto, I started driving Aaron to school again, and continued with my exercises at home. I was doing contract work from home, so I took on less work for a while because typing was still a challenge. About six weeks later, I went back to the gym to do some very light weights and walk on the treadmill. It would take over a year to get back to about 80% of my pre-relapse strength. That was still pretty strong and good enough for me.

Chapter 36

Wedding on the green

—⚭—

"A bride at her second marriage does not wear a veil. She wants to see what she is getting." —Helen Rowland

During the time in Antigua, I repeatedly told Chris that I would understand if he was having second thoughts about marrying me. I meant it. I would have been devastated if he had changed his mind, but I would have understood. His dad had been stuck in a wheelchair for the last twelve years, so Chris knew how difficult life could be when you are immobile. I had been told that there were no guarantees regarding the outlook of my disease progression, but because my first 10 years with MS had been relatively symptom-free, my long-term prognosis had a better chance of being quite good. If that sounds vague, it's because it is. There are a lot of ifs, ands and maybes when doctors talk to you about the future because no one really knows, so I communicated this aspect of uncertainty to Chris.

He listened, but didn't hesitate to assure me he was all in. We moved forward with wedding plans.

Chris and I decided that we wanted a wedding that would include family and just a few friends. Small, intimate, relaxed and warm was the ambience we aimed to achieve. Chris's cousin, Maurice, would stand up for him, as well as be our photographer, and Courtenay was to be my Matron of Honour. Her three kids and Aaron would walk down the aisle together, followed by Caitlin and Stephanie. We knew we wanted the venue to be The Toronto Hunt, a nine-hole golf club situated near downtown Toronto. The clubhouse and outdoor dining area sit upon the Scarborough Bluffs and overlook Lake Ontario. It is one of the most scenic locales in the city to enjoy a meal on a summer day. Sightings of deer, foxes, geese and ducks are common throughout the property. We decided to take our chances with the weather and get married on the lawn outside the dining room, overlooking the lake, on Friday, September 6.

Chris and I agreed that we'd ask his girls to wear dresses in pretty pastel shades that they already had in their closet, he'd wear a new grey suit, pale blue shirt and purple tie, and Aaron and Court's two sons would wear matching outfits. I kept it easy, watched for sales, and ordered it all online. Court's daughter, Sophie, wore a lilac, tiered dress that was cute and comfortable. The kids looked adorable.

Courtenay and I found our dresses in Florida. I was still recovering from my MS relapse and had to conserve energy, so we went to one store that I knew carried lots of white dresses—Court and I found our dresses immediately. I chose a fitted, floor length, sleeveless, v-neck white sheath, made from a large floral lace-inspired fabric. It was well lined, so even though it was fitted and white, my bag didn't show and, with some good underwear, even when it was a bit full, you couldn't see a thing. That was important if I was going to feel comfortable and confident. There were large white lacquer beads framing the neckline, and my upper back and collarbone were exposed, which I liked. I knew that after the wedding, I would have the dress cut short and wear it again many times. That has proven to be true, it's still in my summer rotation. Some things don't change—my pretty had to be practical.

Our wedding day was perfect, with bright blue skies, sunshine, and a slight breeze. I know they say rain brings you luck on your wedding day, but when you make the risky decision to have an outdoor wedding, you cross your fingers for good weather and hope that Mother Nature is on your side. She seemed to want our day to be just right. The wedding planner had gathered our kids, Court, Maurice, Chris, and I to walk down the aisle when I suddenly realized the minister wasn't there. None of us had noticed! It was 5 o'clock and everyone was seated in the garden and enjoying the view of the lake, waiting for us to walk down the aisle. Chris grabbed his cell phone and saw he had a missed call. Traffic was bad and our lady was on her way. I laughed heartily that we had all been ready to walk down the aisle to an empty pulpit. Clearly, no one was sweating the details. Ten minutes later, our frazzled officiate took her spot and we made our way down the lawn.

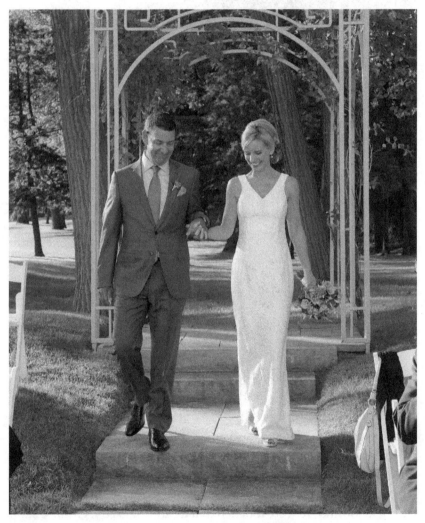

Walking down the aisle with Chris. September, 2013.

Caitlin and Stephanie looked beautiful in their bridal finery. Caitlin in a soft pink, short, fitted dress, and Steph in a flowy lilac dress that skimmed just below her knees. Stephanie plays guitar and both girls sing, so we had requested that they be part of the ceremony musically. For the past week, the girls had been busy practising two songs they were performing before we said our vows. Aaron was only eight

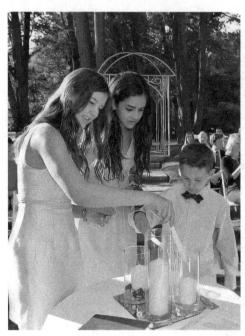

years old, so we had him walking his younger cousin, Johnny, down the aisle, and to their seats, with Liam and Sophie on their heels. Then, after things got started, Aaron joined the girls and us in lighting a unity candle, symbolizing the joining of our families. Afterwards, he happily sat back down in the front row with my parents and his cousins.

Cailin, Stephanie, and Aaron lighting the unity candle. September, 2013.

Chris and I looked into each other's eyes as we said our vows and I felt full of love. It was an emotional moment, and Chris and I squeezed each other's hands even tighter. After we exchanged our wedding bands, kissed and signed the registry, we walked back up the aisle to the band playing "You're the One that I Want" from the *Grease* soundtrack. That was my request, obviously.

Chris and I had planned the dinner with great care. Midway through the meal, Chris's dad, Iain, made a short speech from his wheelchair. This was no easy feat for him because, since his stroke years earlier, when he's tired, finding his words could be a challenge. He did an excellent job and we were touched that he addressed the group. Caitlin and Stephanie spoke next, and delivered their words with their usual grace and poise, with Steph getting a bit teary near the end. Then it was my turn. I hadn't written a speech for my first wedding. I recall being shocked when I was at the podium and realized I needed to say something. I don't remember what I came up with, except thanking everyone for being there, especially the out-of-town guests. For my wedding to Chris, I took great care with my speech and wanted to include our kids and family in my sentiments, as well as letting everyone know how much I valued Chris, our partnership and love. It wasn't long, but I wanted it to be well considered. Chris and I had agreed on five minutes each for our speeches. I had practiced mine and it was four minutes and 55 seconds. All went well and I handed the microphone over to Chris. I didn't have a stopwatch, but as my legs began to ache, I knew he must have been well over the 10-minute mark, with no hint of an end nearby. I moved aside and sat down so I could listen without having to worry about my limbs. A few people giggled as I feigned fatigue, and that was okay, Chris commented that he was taking longer than we agreed. I had white flip-flops in my bag, and as soon as he was done, I put them on for dessert, and dancing. My legs thanked me.

We had a live band, an open bar, and a few more hours until the end of the evening, so after dinner I made it my job to corral people on to the dance floor. Dad got things started with his girlfriend, Lida, and I sidled up next to him, slipping around in my treadless flip-flops. After dancing with us for a while, Aaron started losing steam. It had been a long, busy day. I pointed out two big cozy chairs and a couch just outside the dining room where he could sleep when he felt tired, but he had other ideas. He asked one of the girls to set up two dining chairs at the edge of the dance floor so he could watch, and then curled up and slept when he got tired. The music was thumping, people were twirling and grooving, and my sweet son was happily in the middle of it all, snoring.

I got to talk to and dance with everyone that night, and most of the time Chris was by my side. Just after 12:30 am, as things were wrapping up, Chris scooped up Aaron who was now nestled in my wrap, and the five of us went home to start life as The Ronlands, what we happily called the merging of our two families, the Ronalds and the Irelands.

Chapter 37

Cowgirl

"I am emptier for having lost you, but I became fuller by realizing that losing someone leaves you space to be more of someone yourself." —Craig D. Lounsbrough

When Steve, Mum and I bought our summer cottage in 2000, I always said it would be absolutely perfect if there were somewhere nearby to ride. Five years ago, I discovered a barn about 20 minutes from the cottage and I promptly went to meet the proprietor and sign up for a weekly summer riding lesson. I was elated! A woman named Cindy and her husband, Mike, owned the establishment. They lived on the property, right off the main road, with their menagerie of cats and dogs, most of whom noisily greeted you when you enter the driveway. The backside of their farm faced the woods and an old railway trail that you could ride into town.

The barn was a stone's throw from their bungalow, and 100 yards from there was an outside riding ring, as well as two fenced-in areas to turn out the horses. Cindy had also set up an enclosed mountain trail area to practise going over bridges, wide plank teeter-totters, and up and down rocky hills, among other obstacles for the horses. It was my favourite part of the property because it was so green and full of exciting new challenges to practise. Cindy was an accomplished rider, proficient in both English- and Western-style saddles. With her short blonde hair, tanned skin and strong, fit physique, she was a true horsewoman with a no-nonsense attitude and great down-to-earth sense of humour. She ran a small, humble, casual set-up and I immediately settled into its dusty rhythm and felt at home there. I found a part of myself that I hadn't realized how much I missed, until I had it back.

It had been about five years since I had been on horseback and I was thrilled to be back in the saddle, a Western saddle this time. This old dog had to learn a few new tricks, but the basics were very similar to English riding. I was energized by my time at the barn. People told me that I emanated happiness when I talked about my time there. I felt lit up and apparently it showed.

I used to love when we rode bareback when I was a kid in Vermont. Sometimes, Su and I would ride up from the barn to the main house using only halters with rope as our reins. We knew our ponies, Cheeky and April, were good natured, so we trusted them. We often pretended we were Nancy Drew on a ranch solving a crime. It was fun, but there was another reason why I enjoyed it so much. There was no barrier between the horse and me. It felt so pure, the connection. I didn't want to ride bareback anymore, but still felt the horse's energy as my own. It was hard to explain to people without sounding like a nut, but my MS leg symptoms all but disappeared when I rode, so I knew there was something to what I was experiencing. I use different leg, arm, hand, and core muscles when I ride than I do in everyday life, or at the gym, and my body thrived.

Between swimming in the lake and riding, I felt MS-free. It was a revelation. The psychologist (and family friend) who had employed me years ago at the hospital was a rider, and I told her about what the riding was doing for me. She promptly sent me an article from a medical colleague about the benefits of riding for MS. All my talk of the energy of the horse wasn't just my imagination. There is some truth, and maybe even some science behind it. Also, there is a lot to be said for doing something you love as a means of recreational exercise, especially when you are surrounded by nature. It's healing.

I kept in touch with Cindy and, the next summer, her friend lent me a horse and saddle and I rode about three times a week. I was also asked to join their "drill team" and take part in their musical ride at the annual county fair. There were eight of us on the team, and we had the summer to learn and rehearse a choreographed ride to the country song "Canadian Girls," by Dean Brody. I was a cowgirl for the second summer in a row and revelled in the opportunity to ride every week with an inclusive, fun, energetic group of females, aged 12 to 60, who enjoyed horses as much or more than I do. We did trail rides near the barn as well as our organized practice nights, and I did recreational rides on my own during the week. It was like a dream come true. Aaron, who was nine years old at the time, often came with me to hang out with the other farm animals while I rode. He played with the kittens, guinea pigs, dogs and

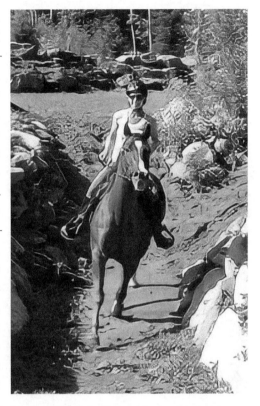

Me enjoying the horse farm near our cottage. Summer, 2016.

goats, as well as tracking the progress of a foal. We bought cat treats at the store so he could "train" the kittens. It was two very special summers getting to share this farm time with him. I felt immensely fortunate, and full of optimism and hope for my health and future.

Chapter 38

My ship is sinking, again

—ᘒ—

"The storm only comes to teach you how to skillfully sail your ship." —
Matshona Dhliwayo

There is nothing much cuter than watching primary school holiday concerts, at least if you are a parent of one of the participants. It's a box full of *adorable*, wrapped up with a bow. In Grade 6, Aaron was in his last year of Junior School, and hearing those scallywags sing always made me grin. Aaron knows I would never miss a concert, and, even though he would say, "You don't have to come, it's *so* boring," I knew he wanted me there.

Mid-December, in the very early hours of the day of Aaron's concert, I experienced an excruciating bowel obstruction. I had been awake and in pain during the night, and my bag had passed nothing since before dinner. Something was blocking my bowel. Chris repeatedly asked me if we should go to the Emergency Room (ER). Even as he clearly started to worry, and badgered me with his concern, I resisted. I didn't want to go unless things got dire because I had experienced two obstructions earlier in my life, and both times, a doctor had to stick something down my stoma to clear the blockage, and one time, I eventually required surgery. I was, and still am, really anxious about anyone touching my stoma. I have been since I was a young kid. The anticipation of it makes me feel like a taut elastic band, ready to snap. I have the irrational fear that my stoma might fall off, and I'll bleed out. I never addressed this in any depth with Dr. Gaze, because it is really rare that anyone gets near me with my bag off. I take excellent care of my health and schedule all my regular check-ups, except with my gastroenterologist, Dr. Greenberg. I hadn't seen him since I had my rectal stump removed 20 years ago.

At five in the morning, after a sleepless night, with me in intermittent agony, I conceded that I should go to the hospital. Chris sent Caitlin and Stephanie a text to let them know where we were going, and so they would be there for Aaron when he got up. I don't remember exactly what we did, but I think Chris called Mum, Dad or Court to come to our house to help Aaron, drive him to school and explain what was going on. In the meantime, I checked into the nearby hospital emergency room, and was quickly taken to an exam room. Chris was with me, sitting beside the hospital bed, holding my hand. After a painkiller took effect, I was able to do some deep breathing and try to relax. An hour or two later, I was wheeled away for a CT scan of my belly. Sometime that morning, Courtenay and Mum came to visit me. I had told them that Chris was keeping me company and not to worry, but they couldn't stay away and I was happy to see them both.

At noon my bag was still empty and I was told that a surgeon would come by and talk to me. I was pleading with myself, please, please, just pass something, even some air. I was being given fluids, so got up to pee. Maybe the walk would get my bowels moving. I tried everything. I asked Chris to rub my back; I moved my legs around a bit, I meditated and visualized my bag filling up. Nothing was working and the pain medications were starting to wear off. I was given another dose. By 1 pm, I asked Chris to send a note to Steve to tell him I wouldn't be at the holiday concert, but please sit with my mum and dad, so Aaron would see he had an audience. We then emailed Aaron's teacher asking him to let Aaron know that he should look for Nana, Grandpa and his dad in the crowd that night. I was okay, but could not be at his concert. His teacher replied quickly saying Aaron was very relieved that I was fine.

After more than 17 hours of pain, I was spent, and almost resigned to knowing my stoma was going to be up for grabs, when I felt a big twist in my belly; I groaned at the intensity. It felt like my intestines were being wrung out. I grimaced, and whoosh, a stream of stool flowed into my bag. I was awash in relief. I think I actually laughed, I felt so happy.

I had Chris hustle to the nurse's station to tell them I didn't need to see the surgeon; my ileostomy was working again. I wanted to get out of there instantly, even though the doctor was around the corner. I barely let him say hello before I announced that my bowels had cleared. He was a nice guy and smiled, said he was pleased to hear that everything was working again, and that he was sure I was happy too. I replied, "Yes, I am, I didn't want surgery, or you messing with my stoma."

He thought that was funny, and had no idea how much I meant it. Mr. Surgeon wasn't keen on me bolting out of the hospital and told me to stay for a few more hours of observation. The moment I received the okay, I filled out the discharge paperwork, promised to book a follow-up appointment with my gastro specialist, then Chris drove me home.

I thought that was the end of that medical blip. After a day or two of taking it easy, my life went back to normal. Nothing changed, although the nasty obstruction did force me to schedule the long overdue appointment with my gastroenterologist. He still had the same secretary, Suzy, and she made me feel a little bit guilty about disappearing for 20 years. I didn't blame her, and felt a bit sheepish, but explained I had been diagnosed with MS and had been having a lot of other appointments. I was scheduled for June, six months away. That was fine with me; it was just a check-up. When I did finally see Dr. Greenberg, he hadn't aged; he looked the same which was some-how reassuring. I didn't associate him with pain. He worked in the hospital where I had my rectal stump removed, but my brain didn't connect him with that period in my life. He asked me some questions about my stoma, but didn't need to see it. He did want to schedule a scope though. I had been worried about that.

I can't have a colonoscopy via my bum, so they have to put a scope down my stoma. I had never had one before and it was partly why I had avoided these appointments. I got a bit sweaty as I explained how nervous I was about anyone getting near my stoma, let alone invad-ing it. I asked if I could be sedated for the procedure. He said yes. I clarified that I didn't want any kind of anaesthetic; I had been put under to have a polyp removed from my ovaries the year before, and

I thought the anaesthetic had brought on an MS relapse. He understood, and we booked a time for the procedure. He also scheduled an MRI. He had received the CT scan results from my trip to the ER in December and he wanted to have another look.

—⚬—

Every year in January, The Royal Bank of Canada (RBC) hosts a one-week Reward and Recognition Caribbean cruise, which can be earned by high performing employees. The bank rents out an entire ship for the event, so it is all RBC, all the time. It's an honour to be chosen for the cruise and people from throughout the organization, all over the world, are recognized, and are allowed to invite one guest to join them. Executives attend with their partners and act as hosts. Chris's boss asked him to be her co-host for the cruise. This meant that Chris and I would be hosting dinners each night for winners, as well as attending social functions on board with the executives and their guests. There are many daily meetings scheduled and keenly attended—there isn't much free time, but people are so energized and thrilled to be on board, they don't care. Forget Disney, the RBC Cruise is the happiest place on earth for the second week of January.

I was excited about the cruise, but as usual, didn't like leaving Aaron. I was also a bit concerned about my health due to the hectic pace for seven days and nights, but was confident that Chris and I would be a good team as co-hosts, and I really liked Chris's boss and her husband. Although I was slightly nervous, I geared myself up for a good week. Chris and I flew to Fort Lauderdale on an Air Canada flight that was filled with mostly bank employees, and then boarded a packed bus headed to the cruise ship. The bus was humming with excitement as people found their spots. It was a big party with people excitedly meeting co-workers from around the country and globe. I hadn't been in my seat for five minutes when my cellphone rang.

It was an unknown number, but I answered anyway.

"Hello, Lindsay speaking."

"Hello, Lindsay, it's Dr. Greenberg. Is now a good time? You sound like you are in a crowd."

I replied, "Now is fine. I am on a bus in Florida. My husband and I are on our way to a cruise for his work."

I had a feeling he had test results for me; I wanted them.

He confirmed this by saying "I'm worried this may not be a good time, I have your MRI results."

I appreciated his concern, but replied, "No really, it's okay. Let me just grab a pen and paper."

I found a pen and the back of my plane ticket and said, "Go ahead."

He began with, "I'm pretty sure you have Primary Sclerosing Cholangitis. I know it's a mouthful so we usually call it PSC. It's a disease of the liver."

I was shocked, "A disease of my liver? I thought the MRI was of my intestines."

Dr. Greenberg explained, "Well, when you had the bowel obstruction and Sunnybrook Hospital sent me your CT scan results, something looked unusual with your liver. I wanted to have another look."

Wait a minute—what? Time stood still for a brief moment and all the noisy chatter around me faded away. I was in a bubble of shock; I hadn't thought that the MRI was anything more than routine. I heard my doctor tell me he was going to refer me to a hepatologist. So far, I had only jotted down PSC and liver. I added hepatologist. I needed more information. I could see Chris was listening to my conversation.

I asked, "I've never heard of PSC, what exactly is it?"

"It's a narrowing of the bile ducts in the liver. It's not a very common condition, but 90% of people with PSC also have colitis/Crohn's" was his response.

I needed to think fast with questions, and my brain was feeling sticky.

I got to the point. "What does this mean for me?"

I wasn't sure I was ready for the answer, but wrote down his response. "Some people could end up with cirrhosis of the liver and require a liver transplant."

Holy shit. I thought, like an old man alcoholic. Is my body confused again by my real age and gender? I think my silence conveyed my distress so the doctor kindly added, "The hepatologist will be able to tell you more. I hope I haven't ruined your cruise."

I replied that I wasn't going to worry too much until I knew more, and thanked him for calling me. I looked at my scrawled notes in disbelief. I had not been worried about my MRI results. I should have asked more questions; I felt like a fool.

After I hung up, I sat quietly and tried to think. I knew that I shouldn't google PSC. I'm not a doctor, and I innately knew that what I might read could be terrifying. Also, if I hadn't had the bowel obstruction and CT scan, I wouldn't have this diagnosis. I am asymptomatic, and that must be good. I was not yellow, or jaundiced, which is often associated with liver disease. I was scared, but I had to be a good hostess for the next week and save my energy for dealing with the cruise activities. I was practised at setting aside my emotions and putting on a brave face, so that's what I decided to do. It was only seven days, and then I could reach out for some support from my family and friends. Chris was holding my hand and looked concerned, but I wanted him to focus on his task at hand. I showed him my notes and told him we shouldn't worry until we knew more.

As we approached the boat, the proverb "Smooth seas do not make skillful sailors" came to mind. The thought of managing another health issue was exhausting. I had a silent pep talk and took a few deep breaths as we boarded the ship.

There was lots going on to distract me, and I managed to compartmentalize my thoughts during that week at sea. I was social and enjoyed myself when I was out and about, but during the day, when the others were in meetings, I went back to our cabin and cocooned in our space. The small area made me feel secure. I read over my brief notes from the bus, cried, and slept. I liked looking out our balcony doors to the ocean, and listening to the sound of the waves and imagining the strength of the currents. I wondered if this disease would shorten my life, and thought about Aaron and estate planning. I planned what I would like for my memorial. I don't picture a funeral for myself. Like my aunt, I wanted a celebration of life. I recalled my happy-go-lucky excursions in Aunt Jill's sports car and singing "Hello and Goodbye." The song's lyrics were perfect for my farewell party: They say nothing is forever, love isn't measurable and the best we can do is make the most of the time we have.

I didn't squash these thoughts; I needed to let go of some of my sadness, or I'd be walking around like an overly stuffed suitcase, ready to bust at the seams, and reveal my private, packed goods at any moment. I didn't want to share my dirty laundry, or, for that matter, anything that I had neatly stored away for the week. I handled things in a way that let me enjoy my role as hostess. I played a mental game. I allowed myself to feel my fear and sorrow in private, and this gave me the headspace to have some fun, and look forward to meeting and entertaining new people.

The first night of the cruise was a dance party. That was a great start, I knew dancing made me feel good, and it also let me off the hook for talking all night. I decided to chat for a while, and then be a hostess that meets and greets while moving and grooving. It's wrong to say that I "decided." I almost feel trapped if I can't move to a good dance song. I need to let my body feel it: I've been that way since my teens, so it's like there's a magnetic force pulling me to the dance floor. Being in the balmy air outside made the crowded dance floor feel open, and I pulsed up and down with the pack and "met" many people that night. I soaked in the energy from the music and fellow revellers; Chris had to drag me off the deck as one of his co-workers reminded us to pace ourselves, the cruise was seven days. I danced my way down our hallway as we made our way to bed. I slept soundly that night and woke early to my husband spooning me tightly.

I was forty-eight years old newly diagnosed with yet another autoimmune disease and, of the 1,800 people on board, only Chris and I were aware of that fact. Along with sadness, I sometimes felt alone. I used my time by myself to plan ahead for when we returned home. I went online and booked appointments with my naturopath and osteopath. I looked forward to their treatments, expertise, and guidance. My friend Angela was a doctor of Chinese medicine—Ang and I had been the best of friends since we were two and a half years old, I trusted her completely. She had introduced me to acupuncture when I was diagnosed with MS, and I knew that I could utilize this to help my liver too. My body had let me down again, but while I spent some time grieving the loss of another bit of my health, I was also using the time to figure out what I could do to combat deterioration.

Six weeks after we returned from the cruise, I went to the appointment with the liver specialist. Chris insisted on coming with me, and it was comforting to have him there to take notes and support me. My PSC diagnosis was confirmed—I now officially had a chronic liver disease. I underwent a liver density test and my score was good (4.4). The mean is 5.6, and it can go as high as 70 in people with severe liver disease. Basically, I didn't have scar tissue in my liver. Furthermore, by looking at the blood tests that I had when I saw Dr. Greenberg, I was told my liver enzymes were fine. Also, the fact that my colitis was stable was good news for my PSC.

I was consoled by the fact that the liver condition was discovered because I had had a bowel obstruction, i.e. it was a secondary diagnosis. My hepatologist told me that because I was forty-eight and had no symptoms, she had good reason to hope that my long-term prognosis will be good. People with PSC have a higher chance of developing liver cancer, so it was now important to have yearly MRIs to monitor my liver/gall bladder to watch out for progression and/or cancer—again, they said, this was not necessarily likely. I would need yearly bone density scans, blood tests, and liver density tests too. None of the required monitoring tests were invasive or painful, so my main concern was finding out if I could do anything with my diet, exercise and alternative medicine treatments to help my situation. I have told very few people about my PSC. It is my third invisible illness.

When I met with my naturopath, Sharon, she assured me that she had other patients with PSC who managed very well. I had been following an anti-mould and anti-inflammation diet for over a year and that was beneficial for this disease too. I wasn't a big drinker, but decided to be even more careful with my alcohol consumption. That was it, what more could I do? As Sharon reminded me, I am a workhorse with regards to taking care of myself. She likened it to "a full-time job," and was confident that I would continue to do the best that I could for myself. I knew I would too. It's the only way I feel some measure of control over my health challenges.

Chapter 39

Nifty at 50

—⟋⟍—

"ILOVERMONT" —Bumper sticker

A lot happened between my CT scan in 2016 and my 50th birthday in August 2019. Caitlin and Stephanie both graduated university, we adopted (and I trained) a crazy little pug-mix rescue dog, Chris and I bought and renovated a new house in Toronto, Aaron completed middle school, and after six months in intensive care and a determined fight, we said goodbye to Iain, Chris' dad. His will to live and indomitable spirit had always reminded me of my Grandpa Ireland. A few months after his father passed away, Chris got a new job that had him in the Caribbean all week, and home on weekends. Five months later, when we had just begun an extensive landscaping project on our house in Toronto, Chris was offered another promotion, this time taking us to live in Halifax, Nova Scotia.

Chris moved to Halifax eight months before Aaron and I. After doing some fruitless house-hunting, Chris and I decided to build a house in Halifax. We had just gutted one in Toronto, so we saved some time and bought a builder's lot. Aaron and I would move after Aaron's school year was over and our new house was complete. We found long term renters for our Toronto house because we didn't want to sell our newly completed "forever home." A big part of the reason that we built a house in Halifax was that I wanted to ensure that Chris and I could still live on the main floor, as we did in our new house in Toronto. I didn't want to waste energy going up and down stairs. MS has forced me to be very thoughtful with regards to managing my physical resources.

I had been going to Halifax every other weekend to see Chris and attend client events. His new job included a lot of socializing and events around town. I finally had the opportunity to wear the black taffeta ball gown that Aunt Jill had given me after holding onto it for 30 years because it was too special to part with. It was perfect for The Festival of Trees, a Halifax holiday event that displays, and then auctions beautiful Christmas trees.

I got ready for the event at Chris's rental apartment, in the very beige and sparsely decorated guest room. As I got ready, I remembered Aunt Jill preparing for big nights in her pink, frilly dressing room. Complete with an ensuite bathroom, huge walk-in closet, four-poster canopy bed, make-up vanity table, and wall of mirrors, it paid homage to all things feminine.

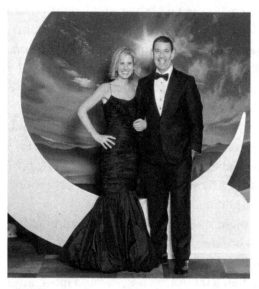

With Chris, wearing Aunt Jill's dress at the Festival of Trees, December, 2019, Halifax, Nova Scotia.

Aunt Jill enjoyed the ritual of getting "done up." She also loved Christmas trees, especially decorating them to exquisite perfection, so being in her dress felt particularly appropriate. I went to more black-tie events during my first holiday season in Halifax than I had in my entire life.

Watching Chris' father Iain fight for his life, and knowing that Chris, Aaron and I were moving to Halifax soon, I became more thoughtful about how I wanted to celebrate my 50th birthday. I enjoyed the parties in Halifax and getting gussied up, but I wanted to be casual for my fiftieth birthday celebration. I wanted something that would nourish my soul. I needed something calm, and to feel cocooned by family. I wanted to blend history with the present. I was craving my roots. I wanted to go to Vermont.

My cousin Val and his wife Shelli owned a house in Vermont. They were excited about the idea of getting together for my birthday. Chris and I rented a house near theirs that would accommodate us, Aaron, Caitlin, Stephanie, Mum, Dad, Court, Brian and Cristina for four nights. I invited my other cousins to come to the celebration. Su already had plans to travel to Costa Rica, but Paul was happy to fly in from Los Angeles.

Besides making sure Val booked a golf game for the men, we didn't do much advanced planning for our time in Vermont. I wanted to visit Uncle Charlie's grave, and go to one of our old favourite family restaurants, Skunk Hollow. Val and Shelli had their wedding reception there, and before that we had many, many nights of raucous fun inside those tavern walls. Su, Court and I would creep around the neighbouring church (where Val and Shelli were married) telling scary stories while we waited for the adults to be done with their dinner. I have memories of spontaneous snowball fights in the parking lot at Christmastime. Aunt Jill would be in her jeans and fur coat aiming snow pellets at Dad, Uncle Charlie and the boys. She and Mum would try and take on the guys, but they were outnumbered, and as soon as the girls heard what was going on, we'd join in to help. After getting soaked with snow, we'd pile in the trucks with frozen fingers, noses and toes, to go back to the farm for hot baths.

When we pulled up at our Vermont rental house, we were immediately taken with its East Coast style. It was a big clapboard house with a southern style wraparound porch, situated on a grassy hill, overlooking the Vermont Mountains. The property was beautifully maintained, with lush white hydrangea bushes in the front yard. The air smelled fresh and pure.

It was a rambling house, and oozed New England charm, with a big kitchen that featured a long pine dining table that suited our needs perfectly. Chris and I went into town to do a grocery shop and I was overcome with how little Woodstock had changed. It seemed symbolic that the lingerie store was gone, but everything else was thriving. The Unicorn, drug and hardware stores, ski shop, jewellers, Woodstock Inn, motel, grocery store—they all looked exactly the same. It felt like a time warp. Forty years later it was as if I was visiting a developer's display model, everything was so perfectly painted and landscaped. I now understood the expression "taking a trip down memory lane." It was a bit surreal, but mostly, the familiarity of it all felt like being enveloped in a warm embrace. That feeling lasted for the four days we were in Vermont.

Our first morning, Dad and Chris prepared our breakfast of bacon and eggs, it's a shared specialty of theirs, then they went with Val to golf. The day was perfect for the girls to curl up on the porch with our morning coffees and teas. We decided on a nearby hike and we all wanted to go into town once the men got back from golfing. I was looking forward to checking out The Unicorn to see if it was as I remembered on the inside, a cornucopia of gifts. Caitlin and Stephanie were interested in finding souvenirs, and we all wanted to visit Quechee Gorge. Now known as "Vermont's Little Grand Canyon," I was interested to see how the area had flourished since we used to visit in the 1980s. Chris, the kids and I walked down to the bottom of the Gorge, sunned ourselves on the rocks, and, after watching another group of kids, Aaron asked if he could come back the next day to swing off the cliff into the deep waters of the Gorge.

On our way back to the house, we stopped in Woodstock to pop into The Unicorn. As we entered, I was awash in a feeling of déjà vu. I had been in this store so many times in the past, and everything was merchandised and set up, as it was when I was a kid. I looked behind the jewelry counter and the owner and his wife were standing there. A genuine Vermont, salt of the earth couple, they had a few more grey hairs, but the way they dressed, spoke and carried themselves were instantly recognizable.

There was something reassuring that when so much had changed in my life, some things remained the same. My history felt intact. It dawned on me then, that this was why I had wanted to come. I would soon be moving to another province, away from my family, and I needed the comfort of revisiting my roots. I instinctively knew I could count on Vermont's stability, and I wasn't disappointed. I felt solidly in the present, but connected to my past. As the owners welcomed us into the store, my mum explained our history with Woodstock. She said, "We used to come here regularly to visit my sister-in-law, Jill Ireland."

The owners broke into huge smiles and said "Oh my goodness, Mrs. Bronson was one of our favourite customers! We used to close the store for her at Christmastime so she could load up on gifts."

I chimed in, "She bought all our stocking stuffers here."

We heard some more stories about Aunt Jill. I had experienced these tales before. Aunt Jill's spending sprees were legendary throughout Vermont, she had a big family to buy for, and she loved giving gifts.

That night, Paul arrived from LA and we went out for dinner at a nearby restaurant that was new to me. It was classic Vermont, with a beautiful garden where we took some family group photos. The inside was like an upscale farmhouse, cozy, with antiques, full of all things past. Chris got a round of champagne and everyone toasted my birthday. I hadn't intended for the entire weekend to be about my 50th, so, soon after the first toast, I raised my glass again to celebrate us all being together in such a meaningful place. Throughout the

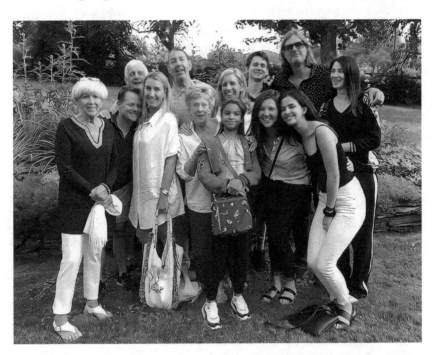

Family photo in Vermont—weekend of my 50th birthday celebration. Summer, 2019.

dinner, Paul and Val regaled us with stories from when they were young, and these tales included my cousin Jason, who died when he was twenty-six of an accidental drug overdose. I liked remembering the three of them when they were young. It was fun hearing about the hijinks that my cousins got up to when they were kids. Su and I had spent a lot of time separate from the boys because they were older than us, so I hadn't known all their comings and goings.

The following evening Val and Shelli were hosting us all for dinner at their house. They spent some of the day preparing, and Court and Bri helped them get things set up. I went back to Quechee Gorge with the kids so Aaron could try the rope swing. Watching the line-up of teenagers and my fearless son plunge into the water, I was reminded of Su. Uncle Charlie had set up a platform with a rope swing at their big pond, and Su loved swinging into the water. I have seen her jump into many lakes, ponds and rivers since. I have to live vicariously through others for this type of fun; the impact of hitting the water would be too much for my ileostomy. I can't say that I care.

After going home and getting cleaned up, we headed over to Val and Shelli's for dinner. I was aware there was going to be a cake for me that night, but that was the extent of what I knew. The evening was gloriously sunny and warm. As we approached their driveway, I saw the garden set up with three round white dining tables and chairs. The tables were set with white linens and gorgeous flower arrangements. A buffet table was at the side, ready for the food, and a catering duo was preparing to distribute appetizers. The scene was so pretty and festive. With Courtenay's leadership, my family had planned and orchestrated a birthday party for me! I felt awed and overcome with emotion. I saw Val and Paul's long-time friend and fellow musician, Rick Davis, setting up a DJ station in the corner. There would be dancing. Rick's brother Davey was also there. The Davis brothers were part of the boys' extended family in Vermont. They all spent hours together when they were teenagers and as they became adults.

I made my way to the entrance to the house, just off the kitchen, and found Val, Shelli, Stella, Court and Brian buzzing around. Everyone was busy unwrapping food and getting things ready. I expressed my surprise and gratitude about all the trouble that they had gone to, to make the evening look so special and lovely. This was the first party that Val and Shelli had ever thrown at their place. Court is a pro at organizing events and had helped them with the details. She had also ordered a poster-size photo of me at one of our recent black-tie galas for everyone to sign. This was set up on an easel overlooking the dining tables. She had hauled all this from Toronto, as well as napkins, stickers, and decorations, all with the theme of "50." She even had a tiara for me, the birthday girl. Silver plastic, rhinestones with pink feathers and a pink 50: I was a half-century princess.

Paul pulled up simultaneously with Jane Ashley and her husband Dudley. Jane had taught me how to ride and ran Aunt Jill's barn when I was growing up. To see them was another fabulous surprise. I was drinking it all in.

The night had just begun, but everything was enchanting. Val had invited his neighbour, and by sheer coincidence, he knew the builder of Chris's parents' house in Vermont. They had sold it years ago, but Cristina, Chris' mom, enjoyed swapping stories with her new friend. The Green Mountain State was a nostalgic place for her too, so this connection made the trip even more meaningful for Chris's mom.

Val, a 6'5" softie, started the dinner with a heartfelt speech. Among other things, he said he couldn't think of a better reason to get together than to celebrate me. He wove Aunt Jill, Uncle Charlie and Jason into his tapestry of words and then he picked up his guitar and sang us a beautiful song. The lead guitar player for Jackson Browne, Val plays masterfully and with his heart and soul. I couldn't have asked for more, but I got it. After the main course, Court stood to toast me, and she brought a tear to my eye. She classified me as her role model, sister and friend. All I could choke out in response was, "Thank you." Later, as I was walking back from the bar, Paul grabbed me to stand beside him as he said a few words. He reminisced about some childhood antics and made us all smile. He joked that he uses call display to vet his calls, but always picks up for me.

Next up was Chris. In my immediate family, I am known for writing rhyming poems for people's milestone birthdays. It's my signature thing. When Chris heard the one I did for my mum's 70th, he made me promise to do one for his 50th. They are supposed to be a surprise, but I swore that I would. Having never been on the receiving end of a poem, and knowing that Chris's forte isn't putting together rhymes, I was completely taken aback when he rose from his chair and read the poem that he had prepared for me. It was very sweet and got a good chuckle. I was touched.

I knew Chris had gone to town to pick up the cake Court ordered, so having the candles to blow out was not a surprise, but the cake was so pretty. It was a rectangular chocolate treat with white icing, decorated with strawberries, blueberries and kiwi. When we were kids, Aunt Jill always threw Su and I a joint party on August 6th, but every year my cake was the carrot cake for the adults, and Su got the chocolate cake. I never complained, but was consistently disappointed. Not this time; everything at the party felt meaningful and special, and it was done just for me.

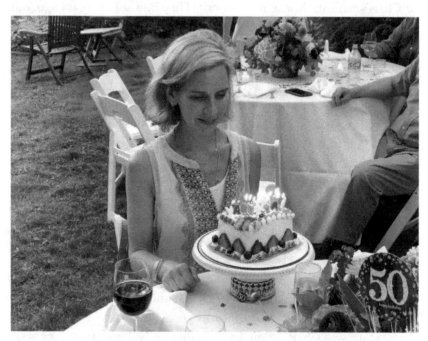

Blowing out my birthday candles in Vermont. Summer, 2019.

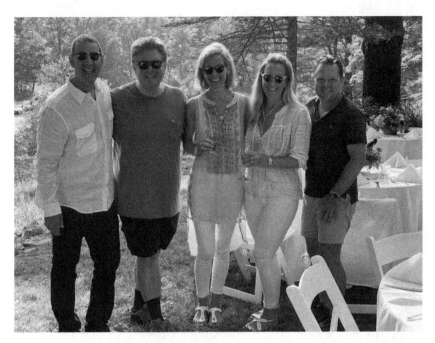

Chris, Paul, me, Courtenay, and Brian at my birthday celebration in Vermont. Summer, 2019.

I got up to thank everyone for the wonderful celebration and the
immense trouble they had gone to, to make me feel fêted. Someone
piped up that they wished Jill, Charlie and Jason were alive to see
this, and I said that I think one of their important legacies is that we
all still want to get together as a family. Jill and Charlie started the
tradition, and long after they are gone, we are lucky to be able to still
gather and openly express our love for each other.

When Aunt Jill died, I worried that the glue that held us together
would be dissolved. Uncle Charlie made it clear to me that it wasn't.
Then, once he was gone, I again thought, without him as an anchor,
we might drift apart. We didn't. It was after her father's death that Su
started visiting me, with her son, at my summer cottage, and I still
connected with Paul and Val. We didn't need one person to keep us
linked, although I was happy to take the lead on plans when I could.
Unfortunately, Katrina drifted away from the family and no one has

been able to reach her since just after Uncle Charlie died. I wonder if she did this for her own mental health. I imagine her role in the family always felt tenuous, because she had never been formally adopted. Maybe it was easier to have a clean break? I wish I could ask her.

It was still bright out when Rick got the tunes started. I don't know if Court had a hand in the playlist, but it was remarkable the way my favourite dance music flowed. Everyone was on the grassy floor shaking their booty. Stella and Shelli were twirling together as Stella exclaimed, "I've never seen my mom dance before." An ex-model, Shelli is tall, rail thin and as limber as an elastic band so I suggested that she break out her moves more often, it suited her. Cristina, usually quite reserved, was coaxed out with the crowd, and Mum, Dad, and the girls needed no encouragement to let loose. I managed to get Aaron to join us and he had a huge smile on his face as he shuffled to the music. Paul and Val were in on the action too. I turned my back on my mum for a few seconds, and in true Paul style, caught him naughtily mock spanking her as they grooved together to a disco tune. Court caught it on video. It still makes us laugh.

I felt so happy that night—really happy. The night had far surpassed anything I could have expected. As the sun disappeared, Stella asked for the floor. She wanted to perform three dances for my birthday. She had taken a few modern dance classes, but was mostly self-taught. She asked Rick to queue up her songs and proceeded to blow us all away with her grace, agility and athleticism. The previous day I had given Stella the magnetic gold necklace that Uncle Charlie had given to me so many years ago. Uncle Charlie was not a verbose man, but he had his ways of letting me know that he cared. Having never met her grandpa, I thought that Stella would appreciate the story behind the necklace and I wanted her to wear it in good health. As Rick shone the spotlight on her, the magnetic gold necklace gleamed and I wondered if my aunt, the dancer, was watching from the spirit world above.

To end the evening, Paul, Val, Rick, Davey and their fellow musician and friend, Kristina Stykos rocked their guitars and entertained us with well-loved songs. Caitlin and Stephanie joined in by performing the Stevie Nicks song, "Landslide." We sat under the moon, in the crisp open air, and bonded through music. When Val was taking a short break, Aaron asked him how many songs he knew. I'm not sure if Val knows the answer to that, but the fact that Aaron asked him delighted me. Aaron isn't easily impressed, but Val had made an impact. My very shy son was trying to connect with my cousin.

The evening had begun at 5 pm, and after six hours, the mosquitoes decided it was time for us to go home. I felt full, and I don't mean with food and drinks. The night had cast a spell on me. I wasn't the only one. Back at our house, our party of 10 all raved about how amazing the night had been. I felt seen, appreciated and cherished. My invisible illnesses didn't factor into any of my thoughts. If anyone had asked me right then to describe past times of feeling scared and alone, I wouldn't have been able to access them. My brain was saturated with love; there was no room for anything else. I wasn't choked up about the goodbyes I would be saying tomorrow, I was too busy experiencing the present like a summer sunrise in my soul.

Epilogue

I talk to my sister every day. When her number pops up on my screen, I know what to expect, a little catch-up call or some venting about this or that. So, when she answered, "How goes it?" with, "I'm in the SickKids ER with Johnny; he has Type 1 diabetes," I was speechless. Literally. There was dead air on the phone. Once I closed my gaping mouth, I managed to ask her to repeat what she had said; I needed to compute it. The news came out of nowhere. She explained that her little nine-year-old son had been tired, hungry and thirsty on the weekend, and over the last while he had been consistently dropping pounds. She never mentioned it in our daily chats because she and Brian had assumed it was due to a big growth spurt.

When Johnny woke up feeling strange on the Tuesday following the "thirsty weekend," Court called the doctor. This happened during the first few months of COVID-19 in 2020, so she found herself talking to an answering machine. Instead of waiting for a call back, Courtenay drove directly to SickKids emergency. Shortly after they left the house, Johnny passed out in the car. Fifteen minutes later, they arrived at the hospital. Her youngest child a dead weight in her arms, Courtenay ran into the waiting room and was admitted immediately. There was no time for panic, questions needed rapid fire accurate answers. Twelve minutes later, my sister was informed that her son had diabetes and might need to go to the ICU. Many hours later, after narrowly avoiding that fate, Johnny was moved to Ward 6A and admitted overnight to be stabilized. A few days earlier, Courtenay had finished reading my draft manuscript. She was spooked by being on the sixth floor of SickKids Hospital. Six A, B, or

C, the letter didn't matter, it felt too close for comfort. It exacerbated her already heightened nerves. It felt surreal to me, so I couldn't imagine how she felt.

Once Johnny's body functions were levelling out, Court called me in tears worried that Johnny would feel invisible and helpless. It was extraordinarily bad timing to have read my story. Our baby of the family was going to grow up fast. He'd have to worry about his health from this day forward.

I closed my eyes and breathed deeply. I needed to mine my composure. I felt like my foundation had undergone a seismic shift, I was off balance, but I found a measured voice as I reassured her that Johnny and I are very different personalities, our diseases are not the same, and that the medical world has gained 40 years' experience in dealing with childhood illnesses since I was a patient. Nowadays there is readily available psychological support for kids and their families.

Johnny has always been a talker and an old soul. He is adept at asking for what he wants or needs. He's insightful, especially for his age, and asks good questions. He's a lawyer, skateboarder, psychiatrist and gamer neatly packaged in a four foot something body with a sense of humour developed well beyond his years. That would all come in handy now.

I told Court that I wasn't going to preach about their strengths and how they would get through this. I reminded her of that by telling her she already knows it. I cautioned her that they were in shock and that shock slows things down so you can work through what is happening. It gives everyone space and time to process and adapt to their new normal while it still feels slightly surreal. I said I was so sorry that Johnny had to deal with this. It sucked. It also sucked that this happened during COVID-19; everyone was already on edge and my sister had to be alone at the hospital with Johnny.

During the pandemic, most hospital rooms are treated like an isolation ward; disinfectant and safety measures are intense. Nurses and doctors are always wearing masks, face shields, scrubs, shoe covers and gloves. Every part of me wanted to be with my sister and nephew.

I wanted to be an octopus and suction my arms around their family of five. Instead, I was far away; the coronavirus made seeing my family fraught with complications. I might as well have been living on the moon instead of Halifax. With travel restrictions and quarantine, hopping on a flight was no longer an easy option.

I kept in touch with my sister via text all day and we were all relieved when Johnny stabilized and was released from the hospital the next morning. SickKids runs an excellent diabetes clinic and over the next few months, Court and Johnny attended many information sessions and learned how to manage his new chronic condition. To say that Johnny has a good attitude about his diabetes is an understatement. During his classroom "share time", Johnny told his classmates about his diagnosis and explained his new illness. This led to many other kids in his class opening up about things they were dealing with. His teacher said it was amazing to watch his young students sharing and supporting each other's vulnerabilities.

Writing most of this book during the pandemic seemed eerily appropriate. As I was documenting the impact of my diseases, aloneness and fear were being felt globally. The power of perspective really hit home. As I edited my manuscript, I realized that my childhood days spent in the isolation ward felt timely now. I documented my past with the knowledge that many people were presently feeling alone and scared. I likened the world to a bunch of isolation wards, except the wards were countries. Things were unnaturally quiet, desolate and sterile. People avoided each other, inside and outside their homes. Strangely, while many people were feeling alone, I did not. This pandemic affected everyone. Everyone on the entire planet. As a child, when I was sick, I didn't know anyone else in isolation. Now, it was the norm.

I felt practised in the feelings; I had been there before, so I adapted quickly. I didn't like the sensations, but was well versed in having limits in life. As I had in the past, I was sure that we would get through the crisis one way or another. It wouldn't be easy, but I buckled up for what was sure to be a constrained existence until a treatment and/or vaccine was found.

I focused on the fact that our parents have their health and adequate financial resources. The same can be said for my sister, her family and my friends. Our family of five all have safe places to live and don't need to worry about their accommodations or where their next meal is coming from. We have green space at our disposal. Aaron, Chris and I have room in our home to spend our days productively, easily. We are immensely fortunate. Watching the toll of the pandemic has been stressful enough, but I knew it could be, and was, much worse for many. It's upsetting to watch the impact on others. There has been so much loss. Maybe that heightened my grief when I learned that Dr. Filler had died in early July 2020.

I knew that I would grieve when Dr. Filler was gone. He had been a hero and comfort to me for such a difficult and formative part of my life. I didn't realize that losing the man that had cut me open so many times, would result in me feeling emotionally gutted. Upon seeing his obituary, my hospital friend Linda and I called each other and wept waterfalls of tears—he had saved our lives.

Dr. Filler kept me as a patient past my childhood expiry date. At one of my last follow-up appointments, he opened the conversation with condolences about my aunt. He had seen the news of her death in the paper and had thought of me. He said he knew how much we had meant to each other. I felt like Dr. Filler saw me and cared about me.

Toronto is a big city, but I ran into Dr. Filler and his wife several times in my adult years. My sister finally got to meet them, and some of their family, at an Italian restaurant. Courtenay and I were there with Mum for her birthday. Mum and I spotted the Fillers and went over to say hello. As I met two of his sons and Dr. Filler met Courtenay—"I finally get to meet Courtenay, I have heard so much about you!"—I saw my mum whispering with my surgeon and his wife. They all looked serious and I knew what Mum was doing. She was telling them about my recent MS diagnosis. I excused myself from my conversation and went to assure the Fillers that I was fine. Five minutes later, after we were settled back in our seats, a bottle of champagne arrived, compliments of the table in the corner. We toasted the Fillers, and then my mother's birthday. Years later, my doctor and his wife met five-year-old Aaron when I saw them at Costco; I told them about my separation from Steve, and, less than two years after that, I introduced Chris as my fiancé when we bumped into them shopping on Bloor Street.

I never got say goodbye to Dr. Filler. Why would I? I was just one of his many patients. Many times over years I thought of writing him a letter. I wanted to tell him how important he was to me. His compassion and ability to make me feel seen in helpless situations stayed with me. He was the one in charge of taking care of my most precarious health situations. He took away my colon, but that gave me back my life.

Like Dr. Gaze, Dr. Filler shaped how I see myself. My relationship with these two doctors transcends me being a patient. They were with me at my most vulnerable and treated me with great care. I wasn't an "easy fix" for either of them. They both made me strong in different ways.

After my surgeries, I used the power of perspective to feel grateful to be alive, I didn't dwell on the trauma. Therapy helped me to acknowledge the suffering that came along with my illnesses. I started consistently processing my emotions instead of internalizing them. That was scary but empowering—I felt more whole and not like separate pieces. It made my point of view more honest, or well rounded.

I value my inner strength, not just in relation to being sick, but as a human being, and, as a woman. I make sure that I am seen and that my voice is heard.

The end

Links

—⁓—

- Crohn's and Colitis Foundation of Canada http://www.ccfc.ca
- Canadian Liver Foundation https://www.canadahelps.org/
- Dr Filler's obituary: https://www.legacy.com/obituaries/theglobe andmail/obituary.aspx?pid=196444872
- Jess Grossman's Uncover Ostomy website: https://uncoverostomy .org/
- MS Society of Canada https://mssociety.ca
- SickKids https://www.sickkidsfoundation.com/

Acknowledgements

—ᴍᴍ—

I started writing this book in 2001 and didn't find time for it for many years. My apologies in advance to anyone I miss in these acknowledgements. I am going to try and acknowledge the people who encouraged me in 2001 as well as the ones who supported me more recently. Some of them are the same, but many are new to my village of supporters.

My heartfelt gratitude goes to the team at WiDo Publishing, but especially, content editor Clarissa Voracek. Thank you for taking me on, and helping my manuscript find new life. You masterfully rearranged things to make the flow of the story more interesting and helped push me to communicate with more depth and detail. You proved to me, once again, the potence of the power of perspective.

An immense thank you to Susan Paterson, for copy editing my original manuscript. Your attention to detail and comments helped fine tune my work. I felt more confident putting my words out there to others once I knew you had gone through them with a fine-tooth comb.

It's been such a gift to connect or reconnect with people through this book. It is with great appreciation that I thank everyone who took time out of their busy lives and read some, or all, of my manuscript (some several times!) and gave me invaluable feedback. Every one of you stoked my fire at times when my confidence and imagination needed igniting. Alphabetical order seems like a democratic way to approach this:

Chris Allen—I appreciate you taking the time to chat about the world of publishing, as well as sending me a list of potential publishers to investigate.

Katrina Holden Bronson—I'll never forget your words "You're a writer!" Your excitement was contagious and gave me hope.

Jane Ely—You encouraged me in so many ways. I can't remember how many times you have read my manuscript, but you can probably recite bits by now! I treasure your loyal friendship.

Kate Fillion—Thank you for sharing your knowledge and helping me rethink my work. You gave me the nudge I needed to make some important edits and keep going.

Jennifer Gillivan—Your response to my book made me cry. I didn't really know you when I asked you to read my draft, but when you shared your reaction, you made me feel very visible.

Stephen Hewitt—All through university, I considered you the ultimate wordsmith. Thank you for your encouragement and kind support.

Jennifer Irwin—I appreciated your keen insights and encouragement after you read my first completed draft. Also, a belated thank you for nudging me onto e-Harmony—that worked out better than I imagined.

Sandy Kellam—After you read my manuscript, your email made me feel that I had an actual book that might be marketable. I needed that, thank you.

Paul McCallum—You read my first draft and told me I had something good to share. I was touched when you called me your "hero" and encouraged me to keep going.

Maureen Reid—Your edits and insights helped make my manuscript clearer and you have been a wonderful sounding board, supporter and friend.

Cristina Ronald—Thank you for your encouragement and helping me imagine my cover design. I greatly appreciate you as a mother-in-law and friend.

Kim Tiessen—You read my very first draft and told me I had a story that needed to be heard. I wasn't so sure, but you were. Thank you for your friendship and diluting my fear about the "poopiness" of my life.

Many people read my book, or connected me with the writer community, and encouraged me to keep going by assuring me that I had an important story to tell. Thank you for your confidence:

Jane-Ann Crombeen, Alison Ely, Lynn Flewelling, Myra Freeman, Leilany Garron-Mills, Steven Laffoley, Bryn Maceachern, Moira MacLeod, Laura Mitchener, Mark Nickerson, Stephanie Nickerson, Brian O'hea, Claire Reed, Caitlin Ronald, Stephanie Ronald, and Becky Skillin.

Dad, in your excitement and pride, you were telling your friends that I was published before I had finished the first half of my draft! You inquired about my writing almost every time we talked and were always helpful in providing me details when I needed them. Thank you for your loving support, it has been inspiring and unwavering.

Mum, your way with words has always kept me in awe. Thank you for being my original editor—you helped me fact check, rethink my format, and persevere. I know how hard it was for you to read some parts of my story, but you kept going, because you believed in me and my work. Your unconditional love gives me strength.

Court, no matter what you are going through, I can always count on you. Thank you for reading my work many times and helping me hash out ideas. I don't know what I would do without you. You are my "sista-friend" always.

Much thanks to my husband, Chris, he has put up with me zoning out for hours while I wrote this book, listened to my endless ideas and prodded me along by touting his pride in my achievement to whoever would listen. He propped me up when I would lose confidence in myself. He makes me feel like I can do anything, and loves every part of me, those are invaluable gifts.

It never seemed to occur to Aaron that I wouldn't be published. He was asking about my book cover long before I was finished writing the book. He wasn't aware how much his blind faith meant. A lot. I am the luckiest mummy.

About the Author

—ᘯ—

To those who meet her, Lindsay Ireland appears to be a vibrant woman in excellent health. However, the reality is entirely different. Despite several serious health challenges, Lindsay manages to live a vital life. When she was 11, Lindsay was diagnosed with severe ulcerative colitis and underwent lifesaving surgery that resulted in an ileostomy. At age 19, with four more surgeries behind her, she set off for university, earning a Bachelor of Science in Psychology.

Strangely, Lindsay's first job in psychology research was in the same children's hospital where she had her five surgeries. Unsettling flashbacks led her to psychotherapy, which took her down the path to self-recognition, insightfulness and illumination. This stood her well when she was diagnosed with MS in her thirties. Since her diagnosis in 2001, Lindsay has been a top fundraiser in the annual Walk for MS, as well as participating in the nationwide Women Against MS (WAMS) luncheon.

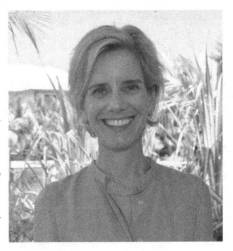

A voracious reader and aspiring writer at the time of her MS diagnosis, Lindsay took a writing course at university and was encouraged by her teacher to tell her story because "it might help others." Writing her memoir became an elusive, but long standing, goal. One of the positive aspects of COVID-19 has been finding the time and energy to write again, and complete her memoir. By sharing her vulnerability, Lindsay hopes that readers will connect with some of the common emotions felt during life's hardships and joys. Connection often leads to empathy and understanding, and the world can always use more of that, especially right now.

Instead of a mid-life crisis, turning fifty felt like a joyous milestone for Lindsay. She continues to find immense fulfillment from her family, friends and community, and is relishing diving deep into her second act.

Lindsay splits her time between Nassau, Bahamas and Toronto, Canada and lives with her husband, son, and crazy little rescue dog, Maxx.

Lindsay can be found on:

- Facebook at https://www.facebook.com/lindsay.ireland.1232
- Instagram at https://www.instagram.com/lindsay_likestowrite/
- Her blog at lindsayireland.com

CPSIA information can be obtained
at www.ICGtesting.com
Printed in the USA
LVHW082356271222
735950LV00006B/92

9 781947 966659